Miss You Already

Living and Loving Through Anticipatory Grief

MEAGAN DAVIES
and STACI FOX

Ballast Books, LLC
www.ballastbooks.com

ISBN: 978-1-966786-99-3

Printed in Hong Kong

Published by Ballast Books
www.ballastbooks.com

For more information, bulk orders, appearances, or speaking requests, please email: info@ballastbooks.com

KEEP THE WINDOWS OPEN

By Natosha Reid Rice

When I think about Staci and Meagan's co-journey through anticipatory grief and their loving, reflective, and insightful book, I am reminded of these words from the brilliant Dr. Maya Angelou, who once said, "I can be changed by what happens to me. But I refuse to be reduced by it." This book magnifies the power of love, the beauty of true friendship and sisterhood, and the need for us to learn practices that can help us hold space for life's contradictions—emotions of joy and pain, laughter and tears, and anticipation and dread—in the face of impending loss and know that they mean we have lived and loved out loud.

I still remember when Staci and I first spoke about her diagnosis. She called to tell me about her diagnosis and to ask me to agree to eulogize her at her funeral. I was taken aback not only by her request but also by her clarity and directness as she shared more about her diagnosis, her reliance on science (some of which, I now know, may have been informed by her many consultations with Dr. Google, as she describes in the book), and her funeral. Wow! I sat up straighter, leaned into my phone, and began asking God to give me the words and the presence to listen carefully and find words that might bring life and encouragement to my dear friend in that moment.

Whew, talk about intimacy. When someone invites you into their interior world while on the brink of life and death, everything else fades away. Staci was center stage. What I sensed in that moment was not an end, but a chance to share life. I heard Staci's voice, heart, and mind, and two things became abundantly clear: 1.) Staci had cancer, but cancer did not have Staci, and 2.) I promised her that even with all the science and medical prognoses, I would do my best to keep the "windows open" for hope and the miracle-working power and presence of a loving God.

Staci has shared her journey with cancer in much the same way that I have witnessed her live—with beautiful honesty, great humor, raw humanity, and now a beautiful haircut. She is a breath of fresh air—a woman who laughs without restraint, is self-possessed, and exhibits a kindness undaunted by the difficult work of pursuing justice for all. When I speak to her and read her amazing social media posts, I am like, how can I laugh and cry at the same time?

Meagan, with her very keen and empathetic insight, skillfully walks us through very tender territory. She handles Staci's story with an erudite pen and a loving heart that overflows throughout. As you will read in this book, Staci and Meagan invite us into the intimacy of their loving friendship, the deep pain of anticipatory grief, and the wrestle of hope and grief, with a determination to live through this journey in ever-present ways.

With its tapestry of stories (as Meagan says later on in the book), this book helps us locate words and ways of explaining and expressing what is often unspoken when it comes to life and death—if we are honest, we are all living to one day die. In this book, as we explore the anticipation of death, divorce, job loss, break-ups, and other shifts and endings, perhaps it will cause us to LIVE and LOVE out loud with a greater presence and urgency. To realize that time is never guaranteed and therefore must be fully realized and lived in meaningful ways.

So, yes, throughout the ups and the downs, the heartaches and pain, the diagnoses, the highs and lows, the fear and the dread, I implore us to keep the windows open—open to allow in light, a bird's song, smells of sweet morning dew on grass, aromas of flowers, fresh air, an occasional appearance of a beautiful butterfly, a calming breeze, and visits from a God who is closer to us that we are to ourselves. May this God open the windows of heaven and pour forth blessings we don't have room enough to receive—a presence with a peace that surpasses all understanding to soothe and heal us along the way.

Staci and Meagan, I love both of you to LIFE,
Natosha

INTRODUCTION

Most of us think of grief as something that begins after a loss—after the funeral, the goodbye, the last chapter. But for many people, grief starts long before that moment. It begins in the quiet hours after a diagnosis, in uncertain hospital waiting rooms, and in the heavy pauses of conversation. It begins when you suddenly see the road ahead and realize, with a knot in your stomach, that you will soon be walking it without someone you love.

This is anticipatory grief, the grief that shows up before the loss. It is the uninvited companion that moves in the moment you learn that your time with someone you love is limited. It is not imaginary, premature, or melodramatic. It is real, valid, and deeply human.

So where was I when I got the call that would change the entire map of my life? I was in Longboat Key, Florida, with my husband, Tim (you'll meet him more fully later). I was standing in the middle of the bedroom where we were staying—a room so large it could have swallowed my own living room whole, easily five hundred square feet of quiet luxury. Everything shimmered in soft shades of gold: the drapes, the bedding, even the light spilling across the hardwood floors seemed touched by it. It was the kind of place you'd expect to see in *Better Homes & Gardens*—elegant, curated, and utterly serene.

Floor-to-ceiling windows framed a breathtaking view of the water, sunlight rippling across the surface like liquid glass.

My phone sat on the side table, plugged in and forgotten. I have a rule about vacations—no devices, no constant pinging distractions. But when I glanced at the screen and saw Staci's name, something in me said to pick up.

It was April 27, 2025.

Her voice, steady but tired, filled the room. She told me she had spent the past few days in the hospital trying to find the cause of her shortness of breath, now made worse by coughing up blood. Then came the words that split my world open:

"I have lung cancer."

The room around me blurred. My body went cold, the way it does on the first sharp, breath-stealing day of winter—when the cold slices through you before you can brace yourself. Shock, fear, and disbelief all collided at once. My heart thudded so loudly I could barely hear my own voice when I finally whispered, "Tell me more."

In the hospital, a variety of tests had been run. Staci's diagnosis was adenocarcinoma—non-small cell lung cancer. It is the most common type of lung cancer found in people who have never smoked. It begins in glandular cells on the outer part of the lungs and is most frequently diagnosed in women, non-smokers, and people under forty-five.

Staci's was stage 4. STAGE 4!

Stage 4 lung cancer, characterized by metastasis, presents significant treatment challenges. It is a sentence no one should ever hear.

Since I was out of town when Staci called, my first instinct was simple: Get home. See her. Hug her. Tell her I love her. And then, almost immediately, came the next question—one that would shape every moment that followed: *How do we support her through this?*

Honestly, in those first few hours, numbness engulfed me. Part of me wondered if this were some cruel joke, a bad dream I would soon wake from. The reality felt impossible.

And yet, reality has a way of settling in quickly. After her diagnosis, every moment seemed to hold a different kind of weight. Ordinary conversations became layered with subtext. Laughter felt sacred. Joy could coexist with a quiet ache beneath the surface—a slow, steady awareness of what was coming.

Anticipatory grief is complicated. And if you're reading this with a lump in your throat, you already know that complexity well. To those of you grieving something that has not happened yet:

- You are allowed to cry into a pillow until it's heavy from your tears.
- You are allowed to be angry, to shout, to throw something across the room, to let the rage burn and release.
- You are allowed to feel relief and guilt at the exact same time.

Your feelings are real. And they matter.

Grief and hope are not mutually exclusive. They can live side by side. You can mourn what is changing while still making space for moments of joy, peace, and even laughter. Both are valid. Both are human.

As Staci and I worked on this book together, we knew we wanted to name the grief so many people carry in silence. Whether you are losing someone to Alzheimer's, dementia, cancer, or another life-limiting diagnosis, this journey demands tools that honor both the emotional and the practical realities. We hope to offer compassion, a bit of gallows humor, and guidance for the road ahead.

If you are reading this, you likely have your own Staci—someone whose presence has shaped your life, someone whose absence you can't yet imagine. You are not alone. This book is for you.

Part I

UNDERSTANDING ANTICIPATORY GRIEF

Chapter One

BEFORE

Let me start by introducing you to the "before"—before I understood anticipatory grief, before Staci's diagnosis, before I had language for the fear living inside my chest. My story doesn't simply begin with her. It begins with the moment my world shifted toward uncertainty in a way I couldn't ignore.

In April 2025, my husband, Tim, and I traveled to Florida to help my dad prepare for chemotherapy for recurrent bladder cancer that had metastasized. Tim and I have built a life grounded in humor, loyalty, and an unspoken pact to shoulder hard things together. He loves fiercely, and that goes for me, James and Maddie (my amazing bonus kids), and our families. Tim is the first person to crack a joke to relieve the tension in a room but also willingly holds me when I cry for no reason. He is the only person I have trusted with my whole heart in a romantic relationship. After retiring from more than forty years in the media business, he took one look at my worry and said, "I'm retired now. That means I can do some of the hard things with your parents. You are not in this alone." I believed him.

We arrived in Florida with a simple goal: to get my dad ready for treatment and stabilize his home environment. But my dad, Stuart, is his own kind of character. A telecommunications consultant in the heyday of the industry, he is charismatic and stubborn and proudly calls himself a "degenerate gambler," spending hours a day betting on horses. He is also deeply resistant to change.

My dad's bladder cancer was back for the fourth time, and this time, it had metastasized to his kidney. The treatment ahead would be more aggressive. At the same time, his wife, Becky—my stepmother—was living with Alzheimer's. She had been diagnosed a couple of years ago, but the disease had progressed rapidly over the last year, leaving my father in the role of full-time caregiver while trying to manage his own disease.

Over the first two days, Tim and I hauled six SUV loads of belongings to Goodwill and the Salvation Army. At my dad's insistence, we took his enormous record collection to a local shop and donated much of the rest to the library, also shipping boxes of Depression-era glass to the National Depression Glass Association. When we finally cleared a path wide enough to breathe, I tackled the pantry. I am not lying to you when I say I threw out more than ten packs of Jello mix that had expired in 1999. Let us not even talk about the condition of the condiments in the refrigerator. I am quite sure COVID may have incubated in the catsup. If you are a full-time caregiver like my dad, you can relate to the fact that many everyday tasks get overlooked due to the time and attention required by the person living with Alzheimer's.

By the time we wrapped up ten exhausting days, both the house and my nervous system were stripped down to the essentials (well, mostly). But to understand why those days felt so heavy, I need to give you more context about what I was already carrying.

To see the whole picture, you also need to know my family's landscape. My parents divorced when I was five. My mom and stepdad have been married for forty-six years, my dad and stepmom for thirty-eight. As of writing this, they now range in age from seventy-five to eighty. Since I was an only child, the five years leading up to my dad's cancer recurrence were relentless. My mom had a stroke and developed a pesky growth in her lung that we monitored with a CT scan every six months. My stepdad was hospitalized with pneumonia, underwent a heart ablation, had a hip replacement, and had shoulder surgery. Did I also mention that he had a bone marrow transplant over a decade ago? Please wrap my people in bubble wrap.

I share all that to say: I was already dealing with a world of shit before I knew about Staci.

On our way back to Atlanta, Tim and I stopped in Longboat Key for a few days of rest. Longboat Key is dazzling: bright white sand; warm, turquoise water; and a kind of quiet that wraps around you like a blessing. After the chaos of my dad's house, it soothed my weary soul.

But even in that beauty, I carried something heavy inside me. A buzzing tension I couldn't shake. A feeling that life as I knew it was shifting. This was the early murmur of anticipatory grief, the body sensing a change before my mind could name it. How did we get here? I am going to let Staci fill you in on the circuitous process that brought her to her final diagnosis.

STACI

I started struggling to walk uphill and climb stairs in December 2024 but didn't think much of it until January. I kept wondering, Am I really this out of shape? *Of course, our society teaches us to blame ourselves for any health issue. One day, walking to the Georgia State Capitol for work, I had to bend over to catch my breath. I knew that wasn't normal and that I wouldn't make it through the legislative session if I couldn't go up and down the stairs easily. It took months for me to get a diagnosis.*

At first, my primary care physician thought it could be allergies, so I was put on an inhaled steroid. Nothing changed, so I went in for an exam. They thought it would resolve, but they also wanted my heart evaluated, so they made a referral. As is common in our broken medical system, it took a long time to get in with the cardiologist. At that visit, I had an EKG and was referred for a stress echocardiogram so they could see the problem in real time. When I returned for the stress echo, the nurse said she'd be doing a standard echo instead. Ugh. I politely explained I was scheduled for a stress echo, and it turned out the physician's order had been misread. They offered to proceed, but I'd have to sign a form agreeing to pay if insurance didn't cover it. I was done. I walked out, called my partner, Greg, in tears, and decided right then to start over with a brand-new primary care physician. That's when my self-advocacy kicked in. Unfortunately, we all have to be our own best advocates.

I changed medical systems and landed in the exam room of the most amazing, kindhearted primary care physician, someone who listened. She wanted me to have a chest X-ray and a cardiac workup. I was willing to start over because I trusted her. While waiting on those referrals, I started wheezing regularly and, during a Human Rights Campaign Board meeting in DC, coughed up a little blood. I contacted my new physician, and she told me to go to the emergency room. I wasn't going to do that out of town, so I cut my trip short, flew home, and headed straight to the ER with Greg after I landed. I'll never forget the date: April 26, 2025. I also need to note that the night before, I was having champagne with my HRC Atlanta family, one of whom has since passed away. I think we should all drink champagne more freely and have more spontaneous celebrations. Drink more bubbles!

I must have been asked a thousand times: "Do you smoke? Have you ever smoked?" Then they suspected blood clots because my chest X-ray was clear, so off I went for a CT scan. I'd never had one before. They injected a contrast dye that made me feel like I was going to pee my pants. Although they warned me, I kept asking, "What if I do?" You have to laugh, even in the midst of fear and grief—another lesson and theme for me.

Then the ER doctor walked in and said, "No pulmonary embolism, but let me show you what I found." On the screen was an egg-sized mass in my lung, and he started using words like "malignancy" and "oncology." I kept thinking, Can't we just take a minute and absorb the fact that cancer has entered the room? *Our friend Liz appeared out of what felt like nowhere to relieve Greg so he could go home for supplies since I was being admitted. In the meantime, I was coughing up blood and tissue. It was really scary. And then there was the googling of "large mass in lung." As good as the care was, I wish there had been more thoughtfulness around even hinting at CANCER. And never, ever spend hours googling your health condition—it's terrifying and hard on our brains and bodies. I sent mine into a tailspin; I was convinced I was going to die within months.*

That night, I texted my sister-in-law and asked if she and my brother could drive my parents over the next day. I knew we needed to see each other and cry, and I knew I needed to say some hard things. My mom sat on my bed, and I told them two things: (1) Greg is in charge, and fortunately, we have a notebook full of all the official documents that we prepared a few years ago, and (2) we are not going to be like Pollyanna; we're going to be real and trust science. We can do those things and still be positive.

On Tuesday, I had a biopsy of the mass. I remember thinking, Where are the female physicians? *And then an angel walked into my pre-op room wearing a Ruth Bader Ginsburg surgical cap. The meaning was already starting to show up for me. My therapist had recommended* Finding Meaning *by David Kessler when I contacted her, and luckily, I'd started listening. It has been such a helpful touchstone, and "finding meaning" has become my North Star.*

Afterward, the pulmonology team explained that while we needed the test results, we were likely dealing with lung cancer. They would be my care team until all the results were back, and then they'd hand me off to oncology. On Wednesday, they decided to do an MRI. I had never had one of those either, and I was alone and scared because Greg had gone home to shower. Also, could somebody please improve that horrid machine? The sounds were so unsettling for me.

The final blow was the MRI results. The PA came into my room, visibly upset; I had bonded with her and with the pulmonologist. (More funny stories, but they're not mine to tell.) She said they'd found a small tumor in my brain. That made cancer stage 4. When I asked, "Will this be the thing that kills me?" her answer was "Yes." Oof.

So we went home to tell our family and friends: I have stage 4 non-small cell lung cancer.

* * *

In the pages that follow, you'll meet Staci, whose story brings this invisible experience to life, more fully. Through her words, mine, and others' stories, we will explore what it means to live fully even as life changes, to keep showing up in love when the ending is on the horizon.

Staci's story is one lens into anticipatory grief, but it is not the only one. As I walked alongside her—and as my own life began to take unexpected turns—I found myself changing too. This relationship and my own experience didn't just shape how I understand grief; it reshaped how I know myself, my calling, and the kind of presence I want to offer others. To understand why this work matters so deeply to me, it helps to know who I was before grief became both personal and professional.

Before I Was a Counselor

Long before the word "grief" took on this new shape in my life, my professional identity looked very different. Today, I am a licensed professional counselor, but my path to this work was not linear.

For fifteen years, I built a career in fundraising and non-profit leadership. I worked alongside organizations that changed lives and strengthened communities. I loved the storytelling, the strategy, and the collective push toward something better. But something in me wanted to move closer—not toward the programs but toward the people. Toward the raw places where transformation begins.

So in 2017, I did the unthinkable: I walked away from a stable, successful career and enrolled in a master of science program in clinical mental health counseling at Mercer University in Atlanta. I was in my forties, sitting in classrooms with people from very different life stages, and yet I knew I was exactly where I needed to be.

Counseling is more than diagnosis and treatment. It is the art of presence, of bearing witness to someone's private world without flinching. It is sacred work. For the past eight years, I have worked primarily with women like Staci—brilliant, capable, deeply driven women who are leaders in their companies, families, and communities. They are changemakers who carry incredible responsibility, often in silence. They keep the world spinning. And they do it while rarely asking for help. When these professionals walk into my office, they are not just seeking therapy. They are seeking permission to be human in spaces that demand superhuman performance. In my office, the mask can come off. The breath can return. The nervous system can finally settle.

Through this work, I've learned that authentic leadership begins with radical self-understanding. This realization shifted my approach to both therapy and leadership. My clients have shown me that anticipatory grief isn't limited to personal lives; it also appears in boardrooms, strategy sessions, and moments of letting go—when a company pivots, when a project ends, or when a dream shifts shape. We will explore this more deeply in the chapters ahead.

I have also been shaped as a leader by the Leadership Atlanta volunteers and board members. It proudly promotes itself as one of the oldest community leadership programs in the country. With a mission to connect and inspire leaders to strengthen metro Atlanta's communities, the program invites participants to look at Atlanta through an equity lens. It asks not just what leadership looks like but who it serves.

That experience gave me language for something I now hold as truth: Healing and leadership are interconnected. You cannot lead people well if you have not learned to hold your own humanity with care. The lessons of Leadership Atlanta still shape how I show up as a clinician, a business owner, and a community member. They taught me that systems heal when people do. Every courageous act of self-awareness ripples outward.

So when I sit across from a client today, I carry with me not only years of clinical training but also the wisdom of a life lived in many chapters: as a fundraiser, a leader, a learner, a counselor, and a human being still figuring it all out. Every piece of that journey informs how I hold space for others. The through line has always been the same—helping people reconnect to what's true, find their footing in transition, and remember that they are not alone in their grief or their growth.

This work changed me long before grief did. It taught me how to sit with discomfort, how to hold someone's story without rushing to fix it, and how to honor the truth of what is. And all of that, every lesson, every client, every late-night paper in grad school, prepared me for the journey I was about to begin. Some of my biggest lessons came from clients. Others came from friends who became mirrors, reminding me that grief and grace often coexist in the same breath.

One of those people was my best friend, Staci.

She is the kind of friend who "sees you." She sees my broken and wonderful parts. She loves me anyway. I found this rare friendship later in life, and when I first learned her diagnosis, it was devastating.

Learning that Staci had stage 4 lung cancer was a punch to the gut, but what followed was quieter, heavier still—the slow realization that our time together was no longer endless. The future I imagined with her was the first thing that shattered. She was my retirement plan, damn it. Both of us have partners who are older than we are, and we have no biological children of our own. (I do have amazing bonus kids whom I love very much). Staci and I had planned to live out our days together with other like-minded women, caring for each other until our own final days.

Staci's story is the heartbeat of this book. She is not just someone I love; she is someone who taught me what it means to live fully in the space between hope and loss. Through her journey, I witnessed what anticipatory grief looks like up close—the courage, the humor, the exhaustion, and the fierce insistence on finding meaning even when the future feels uncertain.

STACI

Hey, y'all! Allow me to officially introduce myself. My name is Staci Fox, and I use she/her pronouns. So I guess I am supposed to tell you about myself. What a hard thing to do. The stuff in your "bio" isn't really the important stuff, so I will give you a bio that goes a little off-script. I am a Sagittarius who was born on the winter solstice. And although I am not into astrology, all the things you read about people of that sign are true about me. I am optimistic most days and passionate to a fault. I can be impatient but flexible, and I am always up for an adventure.

My parents divorced when I was three, and I spent the next twelve years living with my biological mom before running away and ending up with my dad and stepmom, whom I call "Mom." They are two of the most loving people on the planet! In those first fifteen years, I moved around a lot. And that is important to know because I never learned how to maintain relationships.

Instead, I learned how to cut and run, literally sometimes. (Meagan here—I do this too!) *My deep relationships all formed in my adulthood, and some precious ones have endured through all my shenanigans as I learned what it meant to be in a genuine relationship with another human.*

I found the most fantastic career really early. In 1997, I was hired as a health educator at Planned Parenthood in Gainesville, Florida. Inside that organization, I honed my deep understanding of and passion for bodily autonomy. I grew up at Planned Parenthood both professionally and personally, and inside that organization, ironically, my life will end by being robbed of that very thing. There may be another book in me about that.

I was incredibly honored to be hired as CEO by my board in Florida at thirty-five, making me the youngest CEO in the PP world at the time. My final job at PP was based in my home state of Georgia as CEO of Planned Parenthood Southeast and Planned Parenthood Southeast Advocates. And if any of you reading this don't understand nonprofit work, imagine that I was running two corporate entities and three boards across three states—Georgia, Alabama, and Mississippi—in a complex and highly regulated health care ecosystem that was constantly under attack. There is nothing more important to me than this ongoing battle for equity, justice, and liberation.

However, the work at Planned Parenthood WORE ME OUT. I honestly did not know how much until I left. Now, I am humbled to serve as the CEO of the Georgia Budget and Policy Institute. We track how the state of Georgia raises and spends money and conduct research to advance public policies and solutions to address inequities in Georgia. Our North Star is a state budget that centers the needs of those most marginalized by historically racist and sexist systems.

On the personal side, I am partnered with Greg Cole, and we have been together since November 2013. You will see a trend for me. Our relationship was another amazing late-in-life find after many failures for both of us; our theme song could be Brandi Carlile's "The Story." Live music is a big part of our lives. I fashion myself a cook and baker, and my hobby is planning and executing a full meal from cocktail to dessert. Paris is my favorite city, and I bleed red and black for my University of Georgia Bulldogs. And before you ask, no, I never smoked. I have been asked that question more times than I can count. Which made me do this weird virtue signaling at first: "I have non-smoker's lung cancer." My support group set me straight. I needed to check my bias at the door. No one deserves to be shamed, and no one deserves to suffer.

* * *

While her résumé is impressive, what is truly special about Staci is her empathy, her positivity, and the way she absolutely lights up every room she walks into. I found myself dazzled by her at our first dinner together, wondering how to make this human being my friend.

Our first double "date" was at a cozy little oyster restaurant for drinks. It was an Old Fashioned for Greg and white wine for the rest of us—sauvignon blanc, if memory serves. Conversation with Staci felt effortless, the kind of easy that invites honesty. Before I realized what I was doing, I was telling her about my experience with Planned Parenthood during my first year of college. Drinks turned into dinner at a tapas restaurant next door, and somehow, the night unfolded without effort or pretense. I can only remember one other time I've connected this easily with another woman, and that was with my other best friend, Tawnya—whom you'll meet later in the book.

It was at this same dinner that I also got to meet Greg, Staci's partner, for the first time. Greg is also in the nonprofit world and currently serves as the CEO of Buckhead Christian Ministry, or BCM. BCM helps low-income working families in Georgia stay housed and build stability through emergency rental support and financial education.

When I asked Greg what first drew him to Staci, he said it was her "energy, positivity, passion for what she did for a living, and that she was progressive." (*Staci here—My friend Amy said she sold him with my boobs and legs, or so the story goes.*)

During a recent conversation, he said something that stopped me: "The world needs more Staci Foxes, not Greg Coles." I laughed and told him I disagreed. He also shared that her diagnosis made him realize "the depth of [his] commitment to Staci and how intertwined [their] lives are." Knowing them as well as I do, I think the world needs more of both—two people who lead with heart and spend their lives helping others, especially those left behind by systems that no longer work.

As my friendship with Staci grew, we both talked about how difficult it is to make friends later in life and how lucky we were to have found each other. When she was diagnosed with cancer, the news didn't silence her spirit. She brought the same tenacity she used to lead teams and build community into the hardest season of her life. Conversations that once centered on work or weekend plans began to shift toward purpose, presence, and what it means to live while truly knowing your time is limited. From the beginning, Staci faced her diagnosis with a mix of honesty and grace. She didn't shy away from the reality of her illness, but she also refused to let it define her. There were still jokes to laugh at, memories to be made, and lessons to be taught. She let people in—fully, beautifully, and without pretense.

STACI

I want to tell you about Meagan.

You don't usually find a best friend so late in life. Yes, we're proud to say we met in our forties and are currently enjoying our fifties. I first met Meagan's husband, Tim, and he said, "You and my wife are going to love each other." Tim knocked this one out of the park. I don't remember the exact moment we met, but I vividly remember feeling like I'd known this amazing human forever. The bond was instant and quietly strong. Meagan was in the middle of a huge career shift, and I was in awe of her fortitude and vision. I just wanted to snuggle up next to her and never leave.

Although we initially spent a lot of time together as couples, there's never a dinner, an event, or a trip when Meagan and I don't take a few moments to look into each other's souls and listen. Being a woman, being a leader, and growing older have made me value active listening above all. And Meagan always listens.

I also have to tell you about the time Meagan saved me from myself. I am stubborn—REALLY stubborn. It's a survival tactic I learned growing up the way I did. Sometimes, it's helpful; often, it gets in the way of asking for help. In May 2021, I was burned out, broken, and afraid. I had been up all night crying, and in the early hours of dawn, I went for a walk. Somehow, the air helped me gain some clarity, and at 7:30 a.m., I called Meagan and said, "I need help." I didn't know what help I needed, but within thirty minutes, I was on the phone with my therapist, whom I still see regularly, and that afternoon, I was in the exam room of a physician who worked in partnership with Meagan at the time. I don't remember ever asking for help like that before. And I cannot imagine who I would be today had I not called my best friend. I share this because it became a crucial lesson I carried into this cancer fight: I had to be able to ask for help.

So in the ER, when I first saw that huge mass in my lung and the word "malignancy" was introduced, I knew I would need Meagan, and I knew she would respond.

I love Meagan to the moon and back, and this stupid cancer has gotten in the way of our dreams of growing old together, especially since both our partners are about a decade older than we are. So I'm soaking up all the Meagan I can, while I can, and making sure she knows how loved and treasured she is. Because grief is love, and we grieve because we love.

* * *

While much of this book centers on Staci's story and my own, you will also encounter the voices of others who have walked through their own versions of anticipatory grief—caregivers, partners, adult children, and friends learning to live in the tension between hope and loss. These stories remind us that grief, even before death, is a profoundly human experience that takes many forms.

Throughout this book, you'll find reflective questions at the end of each chapter designed to help you pause, process, and connect your own experiences to what you've read. Some chapters will also offer worksheets, journaling prompts, and practical exercises—tools to help you make meaning, find grounding, and move through your own anticipatory grief journey with greater understanding and compassion. I hope that these pages become a companion to you—a steady hand on your shoulder, a place to breathe, and a reminder that even in the hardest seasons, you are not walking alone. May this journey help you discover not only what grief takes but also what it can reveal: your strength, your capacity for love, and the quiet courage that lives within you.

Chapter 2

WHAT IS ANTICIPATORY GRIEF?

Most people are familiar with the grief that follows loss. We associate it with funerals, empty chairs at holiday tables, and anniversaries marked by silence. But there is another kind of grief that does not wait for loss to arrive. It begins the moment we realize that the person we love is dying—or slowly losing parts of themselves to Alzheimer's, dementia, or another life-altering diagnosis. These feelings are common among both caregivers and those being cared for, often experienced simultaneously.

This is anticipatory grief.

Anticipatory grief is the emotional, mental, and even physical response we experience when we know a loss is coming. This unique form of grief unfolds in the shadow of loss, often arriving long before the final goodbye. It begins the moment you recognize that someone dear to you is gradually slipping away. And in the midst of this hardship, life can get interesting.

I'll be damned—sometimes the world conspires to help you. I just picked up a book by Joan Didion called *The Year of Magical Thinking,* a raw portrait of loss and grief following the death of her husband. In it, Didion references Dr. Erich

Lindemann's work on trauma and grief.[1] How ironic that I now find myself referencing the same study she once did. Life is strange that way sometimes.

The term "anticipatory grief" was first coined in 1944 by psychiatrist Dr. Lindemann. Lindemann devoted much of his career to studying loss. He rose to national recognition following his groundbreaking research on bereavement after the tragic Coconut Grove nightclub fire in Boston on November 28, 1942. His findings—from that study and subsequent work—transformed how the medical community understood grief and helped redefine mental health care across the United States. Lindemann defined anticipatory grief as a response to the threat of death rather than to death itself. Those who made it out of the Boston nightclub alive felt guilty for surviving.[2]

The medical community did not recognize grief as a legitimate psychiatric condition. Yet Lindemann's paper "Symptomatology and Management of Acute Grief" would become a foundational document for the standards of psychological care after disasters.[3] He believed anticipatory grief started the moment the hopeless prognosis was pronounced, when the person became aware of the truth of the situation. His research confirmed that the process of mourning begins long before the actual loss.

Why It Is Different from "Normal" Grief

Grief is the experience of coping with loss. It is commonly understood as the emotional response that follows the death of a loved one—the period marked by sadness, disorientation, and adjustment to a new reality.

Swiss American psychiatrist Elisabeth Kübler-Ross forever changed the way we talk about death and loss with her groundbreaking 1969 book *On Death and Dying*. In it, she introduced what became known as the "five stages of death"—later called the "five stages of grief."[4] These stages—denial, anger, bargaining, depression, and acceptance—were initially developed to describe the emotional responses of terminally ill patients facing their own mortality. Over time, however, they have been widely applied to many forms of loss, from the death of a loved one to divorce, job change, and serious illness.

Kübler-Ross's model offered language for emotions that had long gone unnamed, helping both professionals and the public better understand the nonlinear, deeply human process of grief. She later expanded her framework into what became known as the Kübler-Ross Change Curve, a model used across fields—including health care, psychology, and organizational leadership—to describe how people adapt emotionally to change and transition. Below is an overview of how Dr. Kübler-Ross described each stage[5]:

Denial: Denial arises when people resist recognizing the change or its significance. Our brains need time to register a new reality, so reminders of what actually happened may be necessary. As a protective buffer, denial can look like acting as if nothing has changed or hoping life will revert to "before." It can resurface as the situation continues to evolve.

Frustration: As awareness grows, frustration often follows. Irritation and anger reflect the disruption in life and its challenges—but also raise useful questions: *Why is this happening? And how can I cope?* Exploring these questions helps clarify values and begins to guide choices during periods of transition. Values are deeply held principles or qualities that guide behavior and decision-making. They shape motivation, promote fulfillment, and provide meaning in both personal life and work. Making decisions based on your own values ensures that even when frustration bubbles up, your choices remain grounded and intentional.

Staci here: I get so frustrated having to make time for all the appointments. And in the first couple of months, NOTHING seemed to go right. I wasn't eligible for chemo in a pill (stupid genetics), surgery wasn't an option, and after eight attempts to get chemo into my arm, I ended up needing a port in my chest. It is tough to pull myself out of frustration, and then, as most humans do, I end up snapping at the people I love the most. Greg carries the brunt of this, and he does it with such grace. Just this week, I royally messed up my appointments, and luckily, the staff took pity on me and accommodated a shift I needed. My sweet friend Katherine said, "Let's make a day of this," and we went and had a scrumptious breakfast and gabbed and connected all day.

Depression: Low mood can recur. Rather than fading neatly, sadness, hopelessness, or a sense of loss may return—especially as secondary losses or new adjustments emerge. As the impact of the loss becomes clearer, people may experience recurring dips in energy, purpose, or self-worth.

Staci again: Depression shows up for me as loneliness and loss. My amazing therapist, Jenay, always pushes me to use more specific words, usually by sending me the feelings wheel as a gentle nudge that says, "Try again." The emotional fatigue is all-encompassing, and some days, the only thing I can manage is playing games on my phone. It feels like I've lost my sense of normalcy. Yes, the loss of life hangs in the background, but what really gets me are the smaller losses: the loss of some of my hearing and the constant tinnitus (I'm sure Greg is exhausted from hearing me say "What?" every five minutes), the loss of our everyday routines, the loss of our holiday traditions.

This week is Thanksgiving, and usually Greg's mom would be here. We'd spend the week having adventures, exploring museums, and eating incredible food. Thanksgiving would be spent with our chosen family—the Chesters and their whole crew. Instead, I'm headed to chemo today. There's a smoked turkey in the fridge and, my favorite, canned cranberry sauce (don't judge me) waiting in the cabinet for tomorrow. My brain wants to carry on with what we've always done, but my heart feels sad and lonely for all of it.

Experimentation: With some footing, individuals start trying new ways to respond. This proactive phase involves testing strategies, behaviors, and attitudes to see what helps. Experimentation often overlaps with earlier stages and gradually refines coping tools.

In the months after Staci's diagnosis, I found myself trying anything that might help me feel more grounded. There was no master plan—just me realizing that my current strategy of "hold it together with willpower and caffeine" was . . . not a strategy. So I started experimenting.

One week, I tried going to Pilates twice instead of once, thinking maybe strengthening my core would magically stabilize my emotions too. It did not. But at least I could hold a plank without bargaining with God. Another week, I blocked off an afternoon to journal in a coffee shop, imagining myself as one of those serene people who write their feelings in beautiful cursive. Instead, I drank my latte too fast, got heartburn, and ended up people-watching instead of processing my grief.

After visiting Staci during the days of Cisplatin, I also tried taking short runs, which—unlike the latte-induced acid reflux—actually helped. A ten-minute loop around the block gave my nervous system enough time to recalibrate before I re-entered the rest of my day.

Some experiments fizzled; others stayed. That's what experimentation looked like for me: making imperfect attempts to see what helped, noticing what worked, laughing at what didn't, and slowly building a set of coping tools that felt doable in the middle of so much uncertainty . . . but my abs, though.

Commitment and Adaptation: Over time, viable strategies are identified and concrete decisions are made about how to proceed. People commit to new habits or perspectives and weave them into daily life—while remaining open to revisiting, reassessing, and revising as needed. For me, adaptation looked like being worn down enough that I finally surrendered to what actually worked. After weeks of trial and error, I realized that a few of my experiments had quietly become habits.

For instance, I now take a walk or run after every hard conversation or emotionally intense moment. At first, it was an experiment; now, it's practically a lifestyle. My neighbors probably think I'm training for a marathon. I'm not. I'm just trying not to cry in public.

I also adapted by building "recovery time" into my schedule after discussing treatment next steps or physician visits with both Staci and my dad. At some point, I stopped pretending I could go straight from talking about tumors to answering emails like a functional adult. Now, I automatically block off an hour afterward—sometimes for reflection, sometimes for a snack, and occasionally just to stare at a wall and recalibrate. Honestly, it works for me.

And then there's the boundary-setting adaptation: I no longer say "yes" to every request that comes my way. I used to feel guilty about turning things down. Now, I say, "I'm at emotional capacity," which is a polite way of saying, "If one more person needs something from me, I'm moving to a cabin in the woods all by myself."

Integration: Eventually, the change becomes part of the new reality. Acceptance grows, stability returns, and life reorganizes around what is now true. Even so, grief remains an emotional journey; echoes of earlier stages may still arise as people reconcile the past and present, reclaiming a renewed sense of agency and satisfaction.

Meagan and I decided yesterday that we just aren't at integration yet. We've integrated cancer into our lives because we had to, not because it feels stable.

Although anticipatory grief is not formally included in the Kübler-Ross model, many of its aspects still apply. Grief is not limited to death alone—it can accompany any event that disrupts or challenges our sense of normalcy or identity. This includes the loss of defining connections such as a job, marriage, fertility, or a friendship.

While traditional grief follows the loss, anticipatory grief happens in the space between knowing and losing. This timing makes it distinct from post-loss grief. People experiencing anticipatory grief often find themselves rehearsing the reality of death, working toward accepting it, and adjusting to its anticipated effects, all while using the remaining time to resolve unfinished business or say goodbye.

And while all this is happening, the person you love is still here. You can still hug them, talk to them, share meals—and yet you still feel sad. This creates an emotional paradox: joy and grief existing side by side. It is a feeling I know well.

In this space, you might notice:

- **Heightened awareness of time:** Every moment together feels precious.
- **Sudden surges of sadness:** Tears come when you least expect them, even in happy moments.
- **A shifting sense of identity:** Wondering who you will be when this person is no longer in your life.
- **Physical symptoms:** Fatigue, headaches, muscle tension, and disrupted sleep.
- **Emotional symptoms:** Sadness, guilt, anger, depression, and confusing or conflicting emotions.
- **Behavioral symptoms:** Difficulty focusing, forgetfulness, indecision, and trouble keeping up with daily tasks.

Why It's Often Overlooked

One of the most complex parts of anticipatory grief is how invisible it can be to others. It doesn't announce itself, and it rarely looks like the grief we expect. There's no funeral, no obituary, no precise moment when life divides into *before* and *after.* There isn't a sign that you can wear to let people know you are hurting like there is with hair loss related to chemotherapy. Because your loved one is still alive, people may not recognize your sadness. They might say, "Don't get ahead of yourself," or "Focus on the positive." You may even echo those exact words to yourself—trying to stay grateful, trying to remain strong—then feel guilty when the grief still seeps in anyway.

But anticipatory grief is not about losing hope. You can hope fiercely and still grieve. You can believe in better days ahead and still feel the weight of what's coming. Both can be true.

That's the tension of living in the *in-between*—holding love and fear, presence and loss all at once. It's what makes anticipatory grief both deeply human and deeply misunderstood.

For You, the Reader

You may be reading this because you, too, love someone who is dying or slipping away to a progressive neurodegenerative disorder. It can be a spouse, parent, child, sibling, or dear friend that needs your support. The other piece we want you to take away is the importance of advocating for your loved one within the health ecosystem. Medical professionals don't always get it right; that's why they call it "practicing medicine."

When Staci shared her story, I realized something essential about anticipatory grief: It isn't just about waiting for loss—it's about learning to live fully inside uncertainty. Her words remind me that strength isn't found in control or composure but in the quiet courage to stay present even when the ground keeps shifting.

There's a grace in watching someone you love navigate the unthinkable with honesty and intention. Staci's story doesn't neatly tie grief up; it lets it breathe. It reminds us that we can hold hope and fear, laughter and anger, acceptance and resistance at the same time.

As you read her words, I hope you also hear the invitation beneath them: To be gentle with yourself in your own version of "the slog." To give yourself permission to rest when your body says *ENOUGH*, to seek comfort without apology, and to keep noticing small flickers of joy—because those moments, however brief, are the threads that hold us together when everything else feels like it's coming undone.

You may care for your loved one daily or live far away and carry that weight from a distance. Whatever your circumstances, know that what you are feeling is real. Do not shove those feelings down. Your grief does not need anyone's permission. It does not have to wait until the funeral begins. It is already part of your love story.

Journaling Exercise

Spend a few minutes jotting down your thoughts using these prompts:

1. The name of the person you are grieving for now.

2. One specific detail about them you want to remember.

3. One thing you want to say to them while you still can.

Chapter 3

THE MANY FACES OF ANTICIPATORY GRIEF

Anticipatory grief wears many faces, and it does not always look like sadness. Sometimes, it shows up as irritability (I live here a lot—just ask my husband), hypervigilance, or a deep sense of disconnection. Other times, it manifests as urgency—the need to connect, to create memories, or to tie up loose ends before time runs out. What unites these experiences is the awareness that change is coming and that the life you know will soon be altered in ways you cannot fully control or predict.

With Illness

When a loved one is diagnosed with a terminal illness such as cancer, dementia, or ALS, the grieving begins almost immediately—even while that person is still very much alive.

With illnesses like cancer, grief can emerge from the uncertainty of treatment outcomes, the visible physical changes you witness, and the quiet loss of the shared future you imagined together. With dementia or Alzheimer's disease, the grief often comes in waves as fragments of the person you love fade away—memories, personality traits, or the ability to communicate.

With ALS, the losses are often physical first: Mobility, speech, and independence diminish while the person's mind remains painfully aware of the decline.

People often describe this as "losing them twice"—once to the illness and again to death. Anticipatory grief with illness is both emotional and practical: You're preparing for the inevitable while adapting to a "new normal" every few weeks or months. The constant adjustment can leave you feeling exhausted, tender, and disoriented—caught between holding on and letting go.

When David Jernigan was diagnosed with ALS in October 2024, the ground beneath him didn't just shift—it tilted. ALS comes with no cure and a life expectancy measured in years, not decades. The diagnosis forced him into the strange, suspended space of anticipatory grief, where every ordinary moment becomes a question mark and every tradition carries a quiet, private *what if?* Before his diagnosis and retirement, David had served as the president and CEO of Boys & Girls Clubs of Metro Atlanta. Before that, he'd been the deputy superintendent of Atlanta Public Schools. He'd spent twenty-five years doing "purposeful, meaningful work benefitting the children of Atlanta," but that work had left little room for fun or joy.

But this year, even with his diagnosis, he caught himself whispering something he didn't expect: gratitude.

He felt gratitude most vividly as he stood in his living room hanging Christmas ornaments—his "too-early-by-some-people's-standards" holiday ritual. The year before, just weeks after his diagnosis, he had decorated the same tree while wondering if it would be the *last* time he would ever be able to. His body was changing, his future shifting into something he could no longer predict or protect.

Now, he felt gratitude that he was still here—still breathing strongly, still moving (with a little help from a crutch), still able to pull his decorations out of storage and create something beautiful. Gratitude that the ventilator he now used at night had actually improved his breathing numbers. Gratitude that his recovery from a broken ankle was progressing enough for him to walk again. Gratitude, even, for something as sacred and straightforward as standing in front of a lit tree.

That moment of reflection cracked something open. Instead of spiraling into fear about the future, his mind drifted to the people who held him up—his father, his sister, the nephew he watched dominate under the Friday night lights, the friends who showed up in costumes to karaoke bars and birthday parties with deep laughter and bad singing. He thought of the colleagues who had shaped his twenty-five-year career serving the children of Atlanta and of the donors and students who'd honored him in a tribute video that made him cry only once he was safely alone.

In these memories and celebrations, David discovered a quieter side of anticipatory grief—one where sadness sits right beside gratitude and loss shares space with pride. His diagnosis did not take away the meaning he had built across decades: the kids he'd lifted up, the organizations he'd strengthened, the career he'd poured his soul into. Instead, it sharpened his awareness of it.

Joy is simpler for David now. "The things that are bringing me the most joy these days are typically not in the boardrooms or Zoom meetings where I used to spend so much of my time. The things that are bringing me joy are the mornings when I take a little extra time to sip my coffee while taking in the city skyline. Or the nights when I sit on my couch with a bag of French onion potato chips and binge-watch a Netflix series into the early morning hours."

Anticipatory grief often shows up like this: as deep, aching tenderness for the life you're still living but also as fear for the unknown. A sense of time stretching in two directions—backward into everything you've loved and forward into everything you might lose.

Standing in the glow of his Christmas tree, David held both truths at once:

I am still here. Joy and gratitude are still here.

But I know that one day I won't be.

The interview with David was hard for both Staci and me. In preparation for it, we read his CaringBridge site (more on that in a later chapter) and watched a recent speech he'd given. We were in tears before we started the interview. But, as you can read from his own words, we also found gratitude and joy in his authenticity.

In my work and in my own life, I've seen how illness doesn't just affect one person—it reshapes an entire family system. Everyone adjusts in small ways to accommodate new realities. David has seen that happen with his own family as they grapple with his diagnosis. Schedules, priorities, and even conversations shift. There is love in that adaptation, but there is also mourning—grieving the ordinary days that once felt unremarkable.

With Aging

Watching our parents or grandparents age can stir up an entire spectrum of emotions. Although the decline may be gradual, each small change—slowed gait, momentary confusion, a story retold for the tenth time—can evoke a quiet wave of grief. You begin to notice time differently. It no longer feels expansive; it feels fragile and constricted like a shirt that is too tight.

Anticipatory grief with aging extends beyond fearing their eventual absence. It's also about navigating the shift in roles—from being cared for to becoming the caregiver. The people who once anchored you with stability may now depend on you for reassurance and safety. For some individuals, it fosters a renewed sense of appreciation and connection, while for others, it can result in feelings of guilt, frustration, or fatigue. It can also lay bare unresolved emotional wounds that were never tended to.

This form of grief is often quiet and private. There's no diagnosis to rally around, no prognosis to measure progress against. Yet the awareness of limited time is constant. That awareness can spark urgency—to ask questions, record family stories, or create shared memories before it's too late.

As you know, I have four parents who have navigated various medical issues in the past several years. Those issues are also coupled with the plain old aging and the cognitive decline that eventually comes for us. All these events sent me back to counseling. My own counselor is the one who helped me name what I was feeling as anticipatory grief. As my parents began to decline, I started to mourn the people they used to be and had to begin to accept my new role as a caregiver.

I can still feel this loss acutely. And by loss, I mean the shift in my relationship with my parents due to their age and cognitive decline. I close my eyes and cannot imagine a world where my mom is not alive. It takes my breath away just typing that. By the way, as an only child, this part is hard. I am grateful every day to have a partner who shows up for my family and me with grace, kindness, and unwavering presence. My husband,

Tim, is my safe harbor that I work hard not to take for granted as I muddle through these complicated feelings. He is also the person who will crack jokes at just the right time. We were out celebrating his birthday and my mom and stepdad's forty-sixth wedding anniversary, and he told a hilarious story about having to see my biological dad naked after his surgery. "I did not need to see his junk in this lifetime." Yes, these will be some of the real stories you experience on the journey. I promise you no child looks forward to seeing their parents naked as they provide care. But having a good laugh helps.

In our home, Tim and I have created an art gallery, but instead of famous artists, we feature our people and the places that have shaped us. The walls tell the story of our lives—the generations before us and the ones still to come. When I walk past those frames, I feel grounded. I'm reminded that love, in all its forms, outlives loss.

With Non-Death Contexts

Anticipatory grief is not limited to situations involving death. It can arise in divorce, relocation, or estrangement—anytime you anticipate losing a person, place, or role that holds meaning for you.

- **Divorce:** Even before the legal process is complete, you may mourn the loss of shared dreams, daily routines, and the identity of being a partner.
- **Relocation:** A move, whether across the country or across the world, can trigger grief for community ties, familiar routines, and the sense of belonging tied to a place.

- **Estrangement:** When a relationship—whether with a friend, sibling, or parent—breaks down, the absence begins before contact is fully severed. Conversations grow shorter, visits less frequent, until you are grieving someone who is still alive but emotionally unavailable.

In these contexts, anticipatory grief is often unacknowledged by others because there is no funeral, no public loss. This can make the experience lonelier and validation even more critical.

For Sara, grief started in small moments first—standing in the kitchen while her partner scrolled on his phone, realizing she no longer told him about her day, and packing away holiday decorations, wondering, *Whose house will these live in next year?*

Nothing had officially ended, but the losses were stacking up.

She grieved the version of herself who believed this marriage would last forever. She mourned the routines that once felt grounding—Sunday morning walks with the dog, shared inside jokes, the comfort of her husband's body in the bed after a long day. She felt waves of sadness, not just for what was ending but for what would never be: the trips they'd talked about taking, the kids they wouldn't have, and the retirement they'd imagined having together. Gone.

At the same time, she felt guilty for grieving something that hung in the balance, one foot in the shared house and another foot in divorce proceedings. Friends told her to "wait and see" or "stay positive," but her nervous system already knew the truth: The marriage she'd hoped for was over. Some days, the grief showed up as tears. Other days, irritability, numbness, anger, or an urgent need to plan—researching apartments, running budget scenarios, rehearsing the final conversations that would end this limbo. This is anticipatory grief: mourning the death of a shared future while still living inside the relationship.

It wasn't just the end of a marriage she was grieving—it was the loss of her identity as part of a couple, her sense of belonging, and the story she'd once told herself about how her life would unfold. And when the divorce is finally official, people may say, "You're handling this so well," not realizing she had already been grieving for a long time.

Anticipatory grief, in all its forms, is the quiet rehearsal of loss. It asks us to live in two realities at once—the present that still exists and the future we fear. Whether it's illness, aging, or life transitions, these moments invite us to feel deeply and reckon with impermanence.

Chapter 4

THE SCIENCE OF LOSS BEFORE LOSS

The human brain is wired for attachment. From our earliest moments, the brain learns to track and maintain connection—to know who our people are, where they are, and how close they are. These neural maps of relationships are not abstract; they live in brain circuits that process safety, comfort, and belonging. When we're apart from someone we love, the brain preserves connection by predicting if, when, and where we will be reunited. It constantly updates these internal coordinates: *here, now, close.*

These abilities—what psychologists call *object constancy*—develop in early childhood. A baby learns that a caregiver still exists even when out of sight, and this becomes the foundation for emotional regulation. We soothe ourselves by picturing the people who care for us, trusting we will see them again. Over time, our most important bonds become deeply encoded through thousands of loving, intimate interactions, creating an implicit sense that certain people are always with us—even when they are not physically present.

"Our relationships live in our nervous system. They are mapped into us."[6]

Understanding this isn't just an academic exercise. It helps explain why anticipatory grief lands so heavily in the body and why the thought of losing someone can feel like a physical blow. Science shows us *how* attachment gets woven into our neural circuitry; the heart shows us *why* it matters.

So let's shift from the research to the lived experience.

For a moment, close your eyes and think of your loved one. Picture them clearly—their laugh, their gestures, how they smell, the small rituals you share. Now imagine how much your daily rhythm will shift with their absence. There are patterns we build together that become invisible scaffolding of life: dinner at 6:30 p.m., Sunday evening calls, the warmth of a hand in yours before falling asleep. These rhythms don't just live in memory; they live in our muscles, breath, and body. The brain builds expectations around them.

My brain has expectations around my relationship with Staci. I expect good morning texts. I expect we will watch the University of Georgia football games together. I expect that we will go to Highlands, North Carolina, with our partners for Memorial Day. What expectations do you have of your loved one? Now imagine that those constants are threatened.

When that rhythm is disrupted—when illness interrupts the pattern—the brain reacts strongly. The amygdala, the brain's built-in alarm system, flags the situation as a potential threat. It ramps up vigilance, scanning constantly for cues of change: a shift in tone, a missed call, a new symptom. Meanwhile, the prefrontal cortex—the part of the brain responsible for planning, focus, and self-regulation—can feel "offline." Concentration slips. Decision-making becomes harder. It's not weakness; it's neurology.

Researchers now describe grief as a form of *learning*. The brain must literally rewire its internal model of the world. It has to update thousands of small predictions—"They'll walk through the door at 6 p.m.," "I'll call them tomorrow," "We'll watch that show together next week"—to align with a new reality where those things will no longer happen. That mismatch between what one part of the brain *knows* (they are gone) and what another part still *expects* (they should be here) is what drives the waves of grief and confusion.

This is why anticipatory grief is not just emotional—it's physical. It's a full-body response with measurable neurological, hormonal, and physiological effects. When you learn that someone you love is facing a life-limiting illness, your brain interprets that information as an emotional threat of the highest order. In an instant, your entire system is mobilized for protection.

But this shift doesn't happen in isolation. It doesn't stay neatly contained in your mind or your heart. It ripples through your sleep patterns, appetite, energy levels, and immune system—even the way you breathe. Your nervous system becomes hyper-attuned to danger, scanning for signs of decline or bad news. Your muscles tighten, your cortisol rises, and your attention narrows. You may feel exhausted for no reason, wired at odd hours, or suddenly unable to focus on everyday tasks.

Understanding this whole-body activation helps make sense of why anticipatory grief can be so draining. You're not "overreacting." You're not failing at coping. Your body is responding exactly as it was designed to respond when faced with overwhelming uncertainty and the possibility of profound loss. And naming that—acknowledging the physicality of it—creates an important bridge to compassion for yourself as you navigate what comes next.

The Cost of Constant Vigilance

This heightened vigilance can:

- Increase anxiety and hyperawareness.
- Make you more sensitive to small changes in your loved one's behavior or health.
- Keep you in a near-constant state of emotional readiness—an exhausting way to live.

Anticipatory grief often traps the nervous system in a semi-activated "fight or flight" state. You might notice racing thoughts, shallow breathing, tense muscles, an upset stomach, headaches, or disrupted sleep. Physiologically, grief brings modest but measurable increases in heart rate and stress hormones like cortisol, which can impair concentration, decision-making, and memory long before an actual loss occurs.

Your body is trying to protect you. It's alert, prepared, and braced. But that level of readiness isn't sustainable—and recognizing it is the first step toward care and recalibration. This chart outlines the different sections of your brain, how they usually function, and how they react to an anticipated loss.

The Brain's Response to Anticipated Loss

System/ Brain Region	Primary Function	Response During Anticipatory Grief	How It Feels or Shows Up
Amygdala (threat detector)	Scans for danger, activates fear and vigilance	Perceives illness or loss as a major emotional threat, stays on high alert	Heightened anxiety, restlessness, irritability, hyperawareness of changes in your loved one
Prefrontal cortex (regulation and planning center)	Supports focus, logic, and decision-making	Becomes "offline" when stress is high, struggles to manage competing emotions	Difficulty concentrating, indecision, forgetfulness, mental fog
Hippocampus (memory and context)	Integrates memory and helps distinguish past from present	Has trouble reconciling what's happening now with memories of normalcy	Confusion, disbelief, repetitive mental replaying of events
Anterior cingulate cortex (emotional bridge)	Links thoughts and feelings, processes empathy and pain	Heightened activation in response to emotional distress and relational loss	Emotional sensitivity, mood swings, compassion fatigue
Vagus nerve/ parasympathetic system	Calms the body; supports rest, digestion, and social engagement	Becomes underactive due to chronic stress	Racing heart, shallow breathing, digestive issues, sleep disruption

Sympathetic nervous system (fight or flight)	Mobilizes energy to respond to a threat	Stays semi-activated, anticipating crisis	Muscle tension, headaches, rapid heartbeat, fatigue
Endocrine system (hormonal network)	Regulates stress hormones (cortisol, adrenaline)	Chronic release of stress hormones due to ongoing uncertainty	Exhaustion, low immunity, appetite changes, emotional volatility

The Role of the Stress Hormone Cortisol

Anticipatory grief doesn't just live in your brain, thoughts, or emotions—it reverberates throughout your entire body. When the brain detects a potential or impending loss, it activates the body's stress response system as if the danger were already here. This process floods your system with stress hormones, primarily cortisol, preparing you to cope, react, and protect yourself and the person you love. In short bursts, cortisol is adaptive—it heightens alertness and focus, mobilizes energy, and helps you meet life's challenges. But anticipatory grief rarely happens in short bursts. It is chronic, unpredictable, and emotionally layered. The ongoing uncertainty keeps cortisol levels elevated for extended periods of time, which can disrupt nearly every major body system.

Research has shown that chronic stress and uncertainty can dampen immune function, disrupt sleep, alter digestion, and impair memory and concentration, often for months at a time.[7] Studies show that cortisol levels usually stay elevated for up to six months after the death of a loved one, contributing to exhaustion, illness, and emotional depletion.[8]

But cortisol isn't the only chemical affected. Prolonged grief and anxiety also disrupt the delicate balance of dopamine and serotonin—neurotransmitters responsible for motivation, mood, and pleasure. When these levels shift, you might notice less interest in activities you once loved, difficulty feeling joy, or a sense that everything takes more effort than usual.

These changes are not signs of weakness or failure. They are predictable biological responses to prolonged threat and attachment disruption. Your brain and body are reacting exactly as they were designed to—trying to protect you in the face of potential loss. The most often experienced symptoms are:

- **Difficulty sleeping:** Waking up earlier than usual or having trouble falling or staying asleep. *Staci popping in again! Cancer, grief, and anxiety on top of menopause. GIRL! My Oura ring constantly says I am in a sleep deficit, and sleep is at the top of my Maslow's hierarchy. My latest solution is a sound machine. Try all the things: the cold room, putting down your phone early, a dark space, whatever it takes. You cannot tackle hard things without sleep.*
- **Impaired concentration:** Forgetfulness, distraction, or feeling mentally foggy. Grief fog is real, and Staci and I unintentionally proved it. We headed to a women's event hosted by the Atlanta Falcons—a fun, energizing night we'd both been looking forward to. We got dressed, rallied our energy, navigated Atlanta traffic, parked, and walked up to The Gathering Spot, very proud of ourselves for being functional adults. The only problem? We were there on the wrong day. Not the wrong time. Not the wrong entrance. The wrong *day*. Staci looked at me. I looked at her. And then we burst out laughing in that way you do when the alternative is crying. It wasn't carelessness. It wasn't

poor planning. It was our brains doing exactly what overwhelmed brains do: dropping details like they're hot. Sometimes, you just show up to The Gathering Spot three days early and call it a win that you made it out of the house at all. And we looked cute!

- **Lowered immune function:** Increased susceptibility to colds, fatigue, or slow healing. *I'm back! This was like experiencing COVID all over again for me. The mask-wearing, the distancing from others, the incessant use of hand sanitizer, the avoidance of eating in restaurants, and not going to concerts were all reminders—but good reminders. Those things work to keep me safe when my immune system is compromised. My body has changed so much in eight months, and she and I are figuring out how to listen to each other and, most of all, love each other.*
- **Physical exhaustion:** Feeling drained even after rest or like you're running on empty. *I hate this part. I hate feeling tired for no reason, and I hate that society has taught me to think my tiredness means I am lazy. Oh, right, I have a reason, but I hate it nonetheless. I am trying to remember that naps build resilience. I also don't like the assumption from everyone that I am weak. I will ask you when I need you to carry something for me or walk more slowly when I can't keep up.*
- **Mood instability:** Irritability, tearfulness, or sudden emotional shifts. For the past two years, I've lived squarely in irritability and tears. With my emotions so close to the surface, it can take something as small as an Instagram reel of dogs or babies to set off a bucket

of tears—don't even get me started on holiday commercials. I have to work really, really hard not to dump everything on Tim. He's been a trooper, but he's also an easy target, precisely because he's safe.

- **Digestive changes:** Nausea, appetite loss, or stress-related stomach discomfort. *Well, if you are going to read a book about someone with cancer, you are going to hear about lots of uncomfortable things. So here goes my poop story—flip ahead if you want. I had not pooped for nine days. My mom said very sternly, "Staci, go to the store right now and get a Fleet enema." I was willing to do anything to avoid the ER at that point. One of my best friends, Emily, was in town. We'd met in Jacksonville, Florida, through our mutual friend, Kirstin. Emily and I do similar work, so we'd immediately bonded and realized how much fun we had together. Emily had come up to clean our house after my diagnosis. What a gift! So Emily took me to the store, and we bought the "thing." If you ever had a fear of buying tampons or pads when you were younger, imagine buying an enema. So then we came home, and Emily sat on one side of the door while I sat on the other doing the thing. And turns out, Betty was right—it worked. And thank goodness for Emily. It was as close to holding hands through it as we could get.*

Recognizing the sensations described above for what they are—biological responses, not personal shortcomings—can help you release unnecessary self-judgment. You are not "failing" at coping; your body is simply doing its best to adapt to prolonged uncertainty. When we understand these reactions through a biological lens, it becomes easier to see the compassion our bodies are asking for. And while biology helps you make sense of what's happening inside you, it can feel even clearer when you see how these responses show up in real life. So, let's ground this in a real example with Maria.

Meet Maria, a fifty-two-year-old daughter caring for her mother who has early-stage Alzheimer's. On paper, nothing dramatic has happened yet—her mother still remembers most things, still lives at home, still laughs at the same jokes. But Maria's body has already crossed a threshold her mind hasn't fully acknowledged.

Every morning, before she even gets out of bed, she feels a tight band across her chest, as if she's bracing for impact. Her jaw aches from clenching during sleep, something she didn't realize she was doing until her dentist pointed it out. At work, she finds herself rereading the same email three times, her concentration frayed by a constant low hum of worry she can't turn off. She forgets her lunch, loses track of appointments, and startles easily when her phone buzzes—each notification a surge of adrenaline, as if bad news is waiting with every ping.

By late afternoon, her shoulders burn with tension. She keeps rubbing the same spot near her shoulder blade, not realizing it's her body absorbing the emotional labor of anticipating her mother's decline. Her appetite swings from none at all to sudden cravings for sugar. Nights are the hardest: She wakes at 3 a.m., her mind racing through imagined futures—what happens when her mom can't drive, can't remember her, can't live alone?

Maria often tells herself she's "just stressed," but what she's experiencing is anticipatory grief in its most embodied form. Her brain is tracking the loss that hasn't yet arrived, and her body is responding as if it's already happened. What Maria is carrying isn't unique. Anticipatory grief rarely stays confined to one role or one person—it ripples outward, shaping how partners, caregivers, and loved ones move through their days as well.

Staci's partner, Greg, shares the need for vigilance. "I have to be deliberate to stay focused during work. I create tangible goals for each day but give myself grace when I can't get them all done."

He further describes living his life in six-week increments, waiting for the results of the next CT scan to find out if the tumors grew, if they shrank, if more appeared, or if the cancer was status quo, which keeps him in a constant state of worry. Greg's words capture the emotional math of anticipatory grief, the way life becomes measured in scans, symptoms, and small pockets of steadiness. His vigilance is necessary, but it comes at a cost. And while his experience illuminates one version of loving someone through illness, yours may look different.

What you need now is grace—the permission to rest, to feel, and to respond to your body's cues with compassion instead of judgment.

Emotional and Cognitive Dissonance

As we've seen, anticipatory grief activates the body's stress systems—flooding the bloodstream with cortisol, straining sleep, dulling memory, and leaving the body weary from constant vigilance. But the physical toll is only half of the story.

The other half unfolds in the mind, where emotion and logic often collide.

One of the most disorienting parts of anticipatory grief is learning to live inside two conflicting realities at once: Your loved one is both here and leaving. Your days may swing between gratitude and dread, laughter and tears, clarity and fog. This emotional dissonance—holding two opposing truths at the same time—can leave you mentally exhausted and unsure which feeling to trust.

Your mind may tell you to cherish every moment while your body aches with fatigue. You may feel deep sadness while your loved one is still alive, followed by guilt for grieving "too soon." These internal contradictions are not signs of instability; they are the natural byproduct of love existing alongside impending loss.

As a counselor, I talk to clients about "should" statements every day, and they surface often in this kind of grief. "Shoulds" are the quiet rules we carry about how we—and others—are supposed to behave. They often sound like responsibility but feel like pressure. When we can't meet these expectations, they leave behind guilt, shame, or the sense that we're falling short. Most "shoulds" aren't born from our actual values; they come from old lessons, cultural messages, or family patterns we've absorbed along the way. Naming them is the first step toward loosening their hold. The "shoulds" of life can weigh heavily during anticipatory loss, sounding like:

- I should be stronger.
- I should spend every moment with them.
- I should already know how to handle this.

These "shoulds" often come from external pressures—societal ideals about caregiving, family expectations, or imagined judgments from others—rather than from your actual emotional needs. Naming them is the first act of freedom.

Try writing them down. By putting words on paper, you can see these "shoulds" for what they are: external scripts, not moral truths. Once they're named, pause and ask yourself,

Whose voice is this? Does it sound like your mother's, a boss's, a sibling's, a cultural message you've internalized? Recognizing that these voices aren't always your own helps loosen their grip.

Here's one of mine: "I should spend every moment with Staci."

What I've learned is that I need to balance time between caring for the people I love and caring for myself. No decision ever feels perfect. Sometimes, I spend the day with her. Other times, I go for a run or meet a friend for dinner. I've had to learn to live with that dissonance, the ache of knowing that every "yes" to something is also a "no" to something else.

Staci's biggest "should" is "I should be grateful for all I have," which has simply intensified her loneliness. It makes her shut down and not ask for help. *It's true—I find it so hard to ask even when so many people have offered. I don't want to layer on my burdens, and I don't want to be that person who talks about their cancer all the time. And when I need to talk, you never know if someone else is really in the space to listen.*

The key is not to eliminate dissonance but to navigate it with awareness and compassion. Ask yourself, *Does this "should" align with my values, or is it fueled by guilt and fear?* Sometimes, the most loving thing you can do isn't meeting every obligation; it's choosing the action that reflects your capacity in that moment. That capacity may be saying it's time to rest and recuperate.

Reframing helps too. Try transforming "should" into "could" or "want." Instead of saying, "I should visit every day," say, "I could visit today, and when I do, I want to be fully present."

That small shift moves you from obligation to intention. It turns pressure into agency. In grief, presence matters far more than perfection. This process will not be neat or linear. It's messy, human, and constantly evolving. Some days, you'll feel like you're getting it right. Other days, you'll just be surviving. Both are okay.

Since anticipatory grief is not a steady or predictable process, it often reminds us that we are not in control. I know, I know, we all want to be in control. When grief asks for our attention, the most courageous response is to give it. Paradoxically, it's through acknowledging grief that we can create a bit of distance from it. When we try to shove it down and play wackamole, it resurfaces elsewhere—in the body, in our relationships, and in the quiet corners of our mind. If you don't believe me yet, read *The Body Keeps the Score.*[9] You might tell yourself you're fine, but your body will ooze with truth—maybe through a clenched jaw, migraines that flair up during stressful weeks, snapping at someone you love over something small, or waking up at 3 a.m. with your heart racing. When we refuse to connect with our feelings, they don't disappear; they simply look for another doorway out. All of this leaves us asking the same quiet questions: *What's wrong with me? Why can't I just hold it together?*

When grief shows up sideways—through exhaustion, irritability, or a body that won't settle—it's easy to turn on yourself instead of toward yourself. But anticipatory grief is not a personal failure; it's a human response to loving someone deeply in uncertain territory. And that's where the work truly begins.

Finally—and most importantly—self-compassion is nonnegotiable. Let me say that again: Self-compassion is crucial to your mental wellness. The inner critic loves to grow louder during times of uncertainty, whispering that you're not doing enough or feeling the "right" way. Counter it with gentler truths:

- It's okay to feel tired.
- It's okay to laugh.
- It's okay to need space.
- I can love deeply and still need rest.

By combining awareness, thought reframing, values-based decisions, and self-compassion, you begin to release the "shoulds" of anticipatory grief. What remains is quieter but truer—the steady rhythm of love, presence, and authenticity carried into each day.

The Role of Connection

As you start releasing the "shoulds," you begin to create space for rest, for breath, and for connection. Self-compassion doesn't exist in isolation; it opens the door to deeper relationships. When we quiet the inner critic, we make more room for others. The same gentleness we extend inward allows us to show up more authentically with the people who steady us.

Our biology reminds us that connection isn't optional—it's essential. The US surgeon general's 2023 "Advisory on the Healing Effects of Social Connection and Community" named loneliness as a public health epidemic, with health risks comparable to smoking up to fifteen cigarettes a day. The report encourages adults to intentionally invest in meaningful social interaction for at least two hours of connection per day to buffer against stress, depression, and anxiety.[10]

In other words, we are quite literally built to be together. When a connection is disrupted, the body registers it as a threat. But when that connection is restored, even in small, everyday ways like conversation, touch, or shared laughter, the nervous system begins to settle again.

For example, Greg shared that he has "realized the depth of (his) commitment to Staci. Our lives are intertwined, and we are, in the truest sense, partners for better and for worse." Greg and Staci center each other, and that connection is noticeable.

And yet, even the strongest connection does not erase the complexity of anticipatory grief. Love can steady the nervous system *and* bring up deeper fears at the same time. When our lives are intertwined, presence becomes both a refuge and a risk—because to fully show up is to feel how much there is to lose. This is where many people find themselves oscillating, pulled between cherishing what is here and steeling themselves for what is to come.

One of the layers of the emotional roller coaster is the push-pull of wanting to be fully present while also fearing the absence of your loved one. Many people with anticipatory grief describe the tension of enjoying every moment while also bracing for the inevitable goodbye. You may find yourself treasuring a conversation or shared laugh one moment, then immediately feeling dread, worrying about how few of these moments remain. This duality can be exhausting, leaving you caught between presence and fear. Recognizing this tug-of-war for what it is—a natural part of anticipatory grief—can bring some relief. You do not need to resolve the push-pull, only notice it and give yourself grace for existing in both spaces.

After several months of muddling through, with grief buzzing steadily in the background, my roller coaster suddenly plummeted. This usually happens to me when I am tired, and anticipatory grief is wearing me down. It takes more energy just to get through the day. I am exhausted from caring for other people, weary of holding space for clients all day, and tired of not knowing when a loss will actually occur. It is the unknown that is so hard to navigate.

As I write this in real time, I am in the thick of it with both my dad and Staci. The exhaustion is at its peak since my dad is in the hospital recovering from having his kidney, ureter, and lymph nodes removed. While in the hospital, tests showed that he also has congestive heart failure and chronic obstructive pulmonary disease, also known as COPD. While I am in Florida, Staci is still navigating her illness. She has a brain MRI coming up to see if her tumor has resolved or shrunk. My stepfather is having his hip replaced, and my mom is having a device implanted to try to determine the cause of an earlier stroke. I feel hopelessly torn between all of them. It feels like a "lose-lose." This is one of my husband Tim's favorite phrases that I have adopted for my own use. Feel free to use it. He's right—these tradeoffs suck.

I am also crying a lot. I cry when I hear sad songs. I cry when I am alone. I cry when I hug my dog, Cooper. Cooper has been stuck to me like Velcro since all of "this" started. I also cry randomly for no reason. So if you experience this too, know you are not alone. Do not forget that crying can make you feel better because it releases stress hormones, activates the parasympathetic nervous system (which promotes relaxation), and triggers the release of endorphins, which are natural mood boosters and pain relievers. This is what I tell myself when the tears come.

I have never been one to take naps, but this new level of exhaustion often forces me to lie down in the middle of the day. I find myself sleeping for an hour or two. It is what my mind and body require of me. When this happens, I work really hard to give myself grace because I know I am doing what I need to at this moment.

Amid all these complex emotions, joy and grief can coexist. This can feel confusing, even disorienting: How can you laugh while grieving? How can you feel gratitude and despair in the same breath? But both joy and grief come from the same root—love. Allowing yourself moments of joy does not diminish the seriousness of what you are facing, nor does it dishonor your loved one. In fact, those moments of laughter, connection, and lightness can become a vital antidote to the heaviness of grief. They remind you that even in seasons of loss, life continues to hold beauty.

Joy does exist in my important relationships. Greg, Staci, Tim, and I spent a delightful fall day on Saturday having brunch outside at Bomb Biscuit, going to a fabulous British car show, and watching the University of Georgia play Austin Peay in football. Sadness and grief were nowhere to be found that day. While the day was simple, I tucked it away so I could cherish that time again later. That day, the roller coaster was just fast, with no daunting drops or turns. *Staci here. I loved that day! We were all so normal and happy.* By the way, I hate roller coasters, so this season is particularly difficult for me. *Me too! No roller coasters for me—real or emotional!*

Journaling Exercise: Riding the Roller Coaster

Set aside ten to fifteen minutes to reflect on a recent day that was highly emotional. Describe what happened, what you felt, and how your emotions shifted throughout the day. Then, highlight moments when joy and grief intertwined. As you write, ask yourself: *What did this teach me about love? In what ways can I allow myself to hold both grief and joy without judgment?*

With anticipatory grief, the very connections that sustain us can also be the ones that ache the most. The person who used to be your emotional anchor may now be the one you fear losing. My emotional anchor is my mom, and I cannot imagine a world without her. That duality can create deep confusion—the longing to stay close and the instinct to pull back for protection. This push and pull is normal. It reflects your brain's attempt to balance attachment with survival.

This is where relational anchors become vital. Relational anchors are the people, routines, and small gestures that help ground you when it feels like grief is pushing you out to sea. They don't have to be grand gestures or lifelong bonds. Sometimes, they're simple moments of connection that bring you back into your body:

- A text exchange that makes you laugh. (Oh, the memes we send!)
- A walk with a friend who doesn't need you to explain yourself. (Hi, Bentina!)
- A nurse who remembers your name. (Thanks, Lindsey!)
- The gentle weight of your dog's head on your lap (especially my dog). *Can confirm—Cooper is is THE BEST DOG EVER!!*

These small points of contact communicate safety to the nervous system. They release oxytocin—the bonding hormone—which helps regulate heart rate, lowers stress hormones, and restores emotional balance. In essence, connection becomes medicine.

During anticipatory grief, you might find your anchors shifting. The person you've leaned on for years, like one of your parents, may not have the capacity to show up in the same way right now, so you may find unexpected support in new places. This is okay. Relationships are fluid during times of crisis; some grow deeper, while others fall away.

The key is to notice what feels grounding. Ask yourself, *Who or what helps my body exhale?* Those are your relational anchors. Make time for them intentionally, even when it feels easier to isolate. Connection doesn't erase grief, but it helps you carry it. It reminds your nervous system—and your heart—that love still exists in the present tense.

In grief, connection is not a luxury; it's a lifeline.

And this is exactly where science becomes useful. Understanding the *why* behind your experience gives you language for what your body already feels. It bridges the emotional with the biological, helping you see that your responses aren't signs of weakness or overreaction—they're evidence of deep attachment to someone you really love. Science validates what your heart already knows: Anticipated loss is hard because it matters.

I call my experience with anticipatory grief "the slog."

There are days when it feels like my entire body is trying to move through thick molasses—slow, heavy, and resistant. Every minute takes effort. Fatigue wraps around me like a weighted blanket I didn't ask for. On those days, simply existing feels like work.

Then there are other days when I'm training for a ten-mile race, laughing over dinner with Staci, Greg, Tim, and almost convincing myself that everything is okay. Each day feels different, unpredictable, like the weather of my own emotions.

The one thing that remains constant is my fear of the phone. Every time a text dings or the phone rings, I tense up, bracing for bad news. I "anticipate" the unwelcome. Guess what that does? It spikes my cortisol and sends my anxiety soaring. Sounds like fun, doesn't it?

Each week seems to bring a new reason to worry. This week, it was my dad's pathology report, arriving twenty-six days after his surgery. His cancer was staged at T3. I turned to ChatGPT to help me understand what that meant. T3 indicates that the tumor has grown beyond the organ's inner layers into nearby tissues. It's not good news, but it's also familiar territory. We've been down this road four times now. The shock is gone, but the weariness remains.

During that same week, Staci's liver enzymes came back abnormal for the second time, news that could potentially alter her treatment plan and shorten her life. It was a double blow.

That week, I crawled into bed every night by 7:30 p.m., book in hand, determined to hide from the world. My bed became a small, quiet place where I didn't have to be strong. My twenty-five-pound goldendoodle (yes, Cooper!) curled up beside me, his warm body pressed close. He knows when I'm sad. On the days when tears come without warning, he gently licks them away, his brown eyes full of concern and loyalty.

Life has felt hard lately. Heavy. Some days, I just want to disappear for a while, to rest from all the anticipation, all the waiting for the next piece of news. Unfortunately, one of my coping mechanisms is to pull away from the people I love. I retreat into my own thoughts, convincing myself that solitude will help me recover. It rarely does. The longer I stay tucked inside my head, the harder it becomes to reach out. It often takes gentle coaxing from my other best friend, Tawnya, and Tim to draw me back into the world, to remind me that connection is part of healing, even when it feels easier to hide.

But here's what I've learned, both personally and professionally: Grief is as individual as a fingerprint. As you navigate this time, you may find yourself experiencing symptoms similar to mine—or something entirely different. There is no single road map for this territory. The most important thing is recognizing how grief shows up for you, both physically and emotionally.

And because I am forever the counselor, I want to help you tune in to those feelings. Self-awareness is the first step toward self-compassion. To support your own exploration, you'll find a **feelings wheel** in the next section—a tool designed to help you name and navigate your emotional landscape. [11]

Our emotions can't always be fixed or solved, but they can be honored. Naming them gives them shape. And once you name what you feel, you can begin to care for it. As much as I can share what this experience feels like from my side—the waiting, the worry, the ache of loving someone through uncertainty—it's only one perspective. Anticipatory grief is a shared landscape, but we each travel it differently. Staci's journey is her own, and her words bring a truth that only she can tell. In the next section, you'll hear directly from her—a glimpse into what it's like to live inside the story we've been walking together.

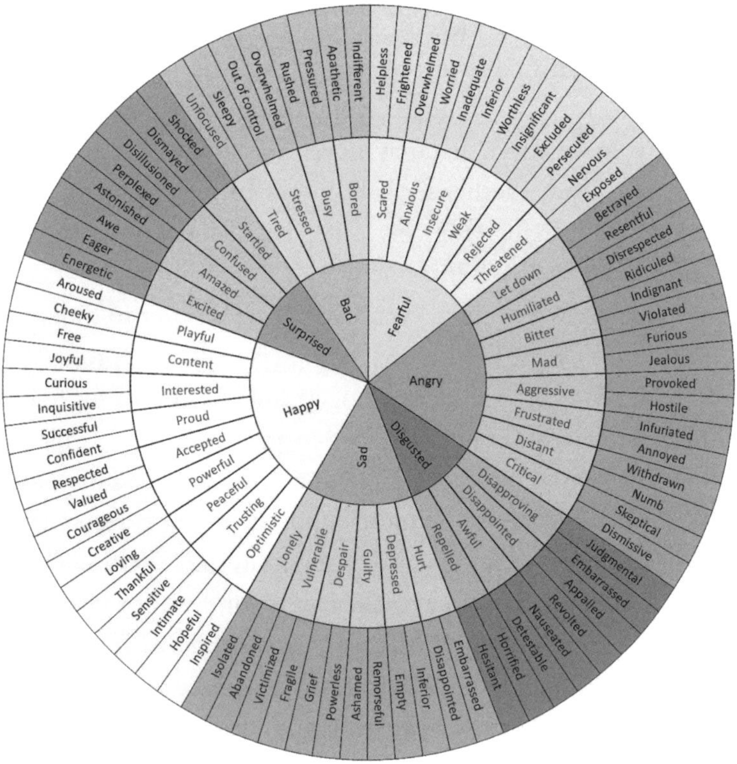

STACI

The first thing I did after my diagnosis was go into planning mode. Before the fear could fully land, I emailed our succession plan to my board at Georgia Budget and Policy Institute and updated our staff. It felt like the only thing I could control: Get the pieces moving and make sure the people I love and the work I care about aren't left flailing.

Then came the late-night scaries. You know, the 2 a.m. Google spirals. There is a lot of information out there, and it can be scary and overwhelming. My first date with Dr. Google was the night I arrived in the hospital. As you can imagine, my mind was racing, and I was trying to be quiet so poor Greg could rest on that pull-out chair thingy. By morning, I thought I had about six months to live and had texted my sister-in-law at 4 a.m. to bring my parents. I had also searched "fuck cancer" and ordered the merch because I LOVE merch. My second date with Dr. Doomscroll was after we got home. I couldn't sleep, so I went to the TV room and grabbed my phone. I started sobbing uncontrollably and finally mustered up the courage to wake Greg and ask for comfort. My best advice is to stay away from Dr. Google!

I'm the kind of person who loves medical stuff and half-believes I am a health care provider after years at Planned Parenthood. But with my own cancer, I noticed I didn't actually want every detail. It felt a lot like stepping away from the horror of the news cycle. You know it's there, but you have to protect your mind. I'm learning to draw a line between "enough information to make decisions" and "too much information to sleep." Seeing the scans changed me. It wasn't just numbers in a portal anymore; it was a picture stamped on my brain. The images made everything too real, and that reality is scary in a way words can't soften.

This whole experience feels like a roller coaster. And as you have already heard, neither of us is a fan of roller coasters. One minute, you might be eligible to get chemotherapy via a pill, and the next minute, your cancer does not have the right genetic markers. Your IV chemo should be easy to get into your arm, but eight sticks later, you can't actually start chemo that day and end up with a port. (By the way, I am SO GLAD I got a port!) One day, your oncologist calls and says he needs to see you that day, and you walk into an exam room to see an exam table and a speculum. Surprise—you are getting a pap smear because they are not 100 percent sure your lung is the origin of your cancer.

Little shifts like those that are happening constantly, just like a roller coaster—no tidy arc, no steady climb. One hour, I think I can handle this. The next, I am bracing for impact. I would like to get off this ride, please.

The Wall Street Journal *published an article a couple of weeks ago about a woman with stage 4 lung cancer, and they used the term "chronic uncertainty."*[12] *Those words perfectly encapsulate how I feel; it hums under everything. How long am I going to live? What will I have to endure? There are many questions and few answers. Cancer treatment and response are so individual. As my friend and fellow cancer warrior says, "We live scan to scan." Right now, I have a scan every six weeks. That really changes your perspective on everything.*

And here's the strange part: Physically, I actually felt better after my first round of chemo because the tumor was retreating from my airway. It felt so incongruent, like my body and my diagnosis were having two different conversations. How could I feel okay and also be that sick? That mismatch messed with my head.

I'm angry, too, specifically at my biological mother for smoking around me for fifteen years. I know anger doesn't rewind time or undo exposure, but it shows up.

The FATIGUE is real. It is as if someone turned gravity up a notch. I'll start a sentence and forget where it was going, open a book and read the same paragraph three times, or just stare at my work to-do list. Nausea doesn't just make you sick; it shrinks your world. I hate it. It steals simple pleasures and makes the days feel smaller.

And then there's the loss of joy. My mouth tasted like garbage while I was on the heavy chemo, so nothing I ate or drank tasted good. Not Dr. Pepper Zero, not a pink lady apple, not even a piece of caramel. And I love to cook. It is my therapy to plan and execute a meal, but it was like someone had turned down the saturation and richness of my life. Joy used to be easy; now it's something I have to look for on purpose. And I just want a margarita!

So yes, I made a plan. I set boundaries with information. I rode (and am riding) the roller coaster. I got mad. I got scared. I got tired, so tired. And I'm learning that I can contain all of this at once: the parts of me that keep moving, the parts that need to curl up, and the parts that, somehow, still manage to hope.

Practical Takeaway

When you feel your anxiety rising or your mood shifting quickly, pause and remember: *My brain is protecting me from loss it knows is coming.* This is not weakness—it is wiring.

Journaling Exercise

1. Where do I feel grief in my body today (tight chest, stomach, jaw)? What was the cue?

2. Which daily events keep me waiting for my person (texts, coffee, evening check-ins)? What can I do for myself in these moments?

3. When does sadness or loss surge? What do I tend to do next—and what could soothe me in these moments (call a friend, step outside, hold a keepsake)?

4. What is one simple ritual I can use on hard days or clinic/hospital days?

Worksheet for "Shoulds"

A Reflection + Reframing Worksheet

Anticipatory grief often brings a flood of "shoulds"—voices of guilt, obligation, or outside expectations. This worksheet will help you name them, explore where they come from, and reframe them into more compassionate choices.

Step 1: Identify Your "Shoulds"

Write down the most common "should" thoughts that come up for you in this season.

Examples:

- I should be stronger.
- I should visit every day.
- I should never feel tired.
- I should be grateful, not sad.

My "Shoulds"

1.
2.
3.
4.
5.

Step 2: Whose Voice Is It?

For each "should," ask yourself, *Where did this come from?* Sometimes, these beliefs come from family, culture, church, or even our own inner critic. Naming the source helps you see the difference between external pressure and your actual needs.

My "Should"	Whose Voice Is This?	Does This Align with My Values?
Example: I should visit every day.	My siblings' expectations.	Sometimes, but not always. Quality matters more than quantity for me.

Step 3: Reframe the "Should"

Replace "should" with "could" or "want." This simple language shift transforms pressure into a choice.

Examples:

- "I should be stronger." → "I could allow myself to rest because strength includes knowing my limits."
- "I should visit every day" → "I want to visit when I can be present, even if that's not every day."

My Reframes

1.
2.
3.
4.
5.

Step 4: Practice Self-Compassion

Write a gentle statement to yourself that acknowledges both grief and your humanity.

Examples:

- "It's okay to feel tired."
- "I can take a break from caregiving to recharge."
- "Joy and grief can live side by side."

My Compassionate Reminders

1.
2.
3.
4.
5.

Final Reflection

- Which "should" feels heaviest right now?

- What happens in your body when you reframe it into a "could" or "want"?

- What would it look like to honor your values instead of giving in to the pressure of "shoulds"?

Remember: Anticipatory grief is heavy enough on its own. Releasing the "shoulds" is not about doing more—it is about freeing yourself to grieve and love authentically, with compassion for yourself in the process.

Journaling Exercise

- Who or what are you currently anticipating losing?

- Is this loss tied to illness, aging, or a non-death life change?

- How is this anticipation affecting the way you relate to the person, place, or role?

- What feelings arise when you think about change—sadness, guilt, relief, or something else?

- Are you withdrawing to protect yourself from pain, or are you leaning in to make the most of the remaining time?

- How could naming the loss to yourself—or to someone you trust—shift your experience of it?

Part II

LIVING IN THE "IN-BETWEEN"

CHAPTER 5

RELATIONSHIPS UNDER PRESSURE

Relationships and mental health are tightly intertwined. They can buffer stress and foster resilience or amplify anxiety, depression, and burnout. During highly emotional periods—such as serious illness, caregiving, job loss, conflict, or grief—relationships are often stretched to their limits. Communication patterns, attachment styles, and boundaries become especially important. Clear requests for support, predictable routines, and shared problem-solving can protect well-being, while avoidance, criticism, or role overload can worsen symptoms. In practice, this means you must tend to the relationship.

What does that mean? It means listening, naming needs, setting limits, and making repairs after conflict. In the middle of all this uncertainty, the smallest conversations can carry an outsized emotional charge, which is why it helps to name what supports connection—and what shuts it down.

As Staci and I have been on our journey, we've seen first-hand how relationships shift for the better and for the worse. Our goal is to give guidance on how to show up as a good human being in times of stress.

What Not to Say

When someone we love is facing a life-limiting diagnosis, conversations take on a new weight. Words that once flowed easily can suddenly feel impossible—too trivial, too heavy, or too risky. In these moments, many people struggle with what to say, what not to say, and how to set boundaries as roles and relationships shift.

This chapter is meant to be a guide for navigating these conversations with compassion and honesty. My favorite saying is "Clear is kind," thanks to Brené Brown.

In moments of fear and sadness, grief needs presence. It asks for listening, validation, and practical support—not solutions. You don't have to "fix" anything. People often reach for clichés, empty reassurances, or quick fixes—anything to soften the edges of pain. It's not usually malicious—it's discomfort. Most of us were never taught how to sit with grief, so we scramble to make it smaller, tidier, or more "positive." We default to statements that minimize ("It's God's will"), compare ("At least . . ."), spiritualize prematurely ("They're going to a better place"), or redirect the focus back to ourselves. While well-intentioned, these phrases can land with a thud, leaving the grieving person feeling unseen, isolated, or even ashamed for hurting "too much." With that in mind, here are a few of my favorite cringeworthy responses and why they miss the mark:

- "Everything happens for a reason."
- "Stay strong."
- "At least you've had time together."
- "You'll get through this."

- "I don't need to hear your cancer story."
- "We could all die tomorrow."
- "God will heal you."

JUST DON'T SAY THESE THINGS!

These statements often minimize the reality of pain by offering quick comfort instead of honest acknowledgment. Though well-intentioned, they can inadvertently signal that the grief is too uncomfortable to face out loud, leaving the person you care about feeling dismissed, silenced, or even guilty for hurting. Rather than making room for vulnerability, these phrases imply that hard emotions should be managed, hidden, or "fixed." That message deepens isolation at the very moment when connection matters most.

When I asked Greg what comments had landed poorly during Staci's illness, he didn't hesitate. Two stood out: "I know that God is going to heal her" and "Wishing you a complete and speedy recovery." He explained that statements like these carry assumptions that can feel dismissive or theologically misguided. "God doesn't choose to heal some people and not others," he said. "That's just not a sound theological position." As a former Episcopal priest, he speaks from years of pastoral experience and from the raw, personal truth of loving someone through uncertainty.

Staci here. Lately, I have learned to detest the "You look great" comments or the mentions to someone else that I "don't look sick." No one knows what another human is carrying. I do not need to apologize for not looking sicker. And we are way too focused on looks anyway. Just say, "It is great to see you." I find myself talking about my cancer, feelings, and thoughts as much as I want. I do not have time to do the work of making other people comfortable; it's hard enough to do that for myself. And for me, hearing about someone else's cancer experience in response to mine is not helpful; it is not empathy.

Preach, Staci!

It's completely normal to feel awkward or unsure around someone who is dying or living with a serious illness, even when that person is someone you love deeply. We often fear saying the wrong thing or worry that we might make the situation worse. There's also the quiet anxiety that our loved one might cry or express pain, and we won't know how to comfort them. These fears are human; they come from our wish to protect both ourselves and the person we care about from further hurt.

The good news is that we can learn to show up differently. By choosing words that acknowledge rather than avoid the circumstances, we can create space for truth and tenderness. I have put together some examples of how to reframe common and well-meaning but unhelpful sayings into ones that offer genuine presence and compassion.

Reframing Unhelpful Phrases

"Everything happens for a reason."

- **Why it hurts:** Suggests that suffering is justified or purposeful, which can feel dismissive when someone is in deep pain.
- **Try this instead:** "I don't have answers for why this is happening, but I want to be here with you through it."

"Stay strong."

- **Why it hurts:** Implies that showing emotions is a weakness and discourages vulnerability at a time when it's most healing.
- **Try this instead:** "It's okay to feel everything you're feeling. You don't have to carry this alone."

"At least you've had time together."

- **Why it hurts:** Uses comparison to soften the loss but can instead invalidate the depth of their grief and longing.
- **Try this instead:** "I know how much this time together has meant. How can I help you make sure you get the time you need?" or "What memories are standing out to you right now?"

"You'll get through this."

- **Why it hurts:** Pushes the person toward a future outcome instead of honoring their present pain, which can feel rushed or dismissive.
- **Try this instead:** "This is so hard. How are you getting through today?"

What to Say

I just gave you some examples of how to reframe these important conversations in a much more empathetic way. Choose words that validate, acknowledge, and invite openness. A simple, heartfelt response is often best. Here are a few examples that you can add to your repertoire.

- "I don't know what to say, but I'm here with you."
- "This must be so hard. How are you feeling today?"
- "I'm holding space for whatever you need right now."
- "Would you like to talk about it, or would you prefer some quiet company?"
- "Can I bring you dinner tonight, do your grocery shopping, or just hang out tonight?"

It's less about finding the *perfect* words and more about showing up authentically. This may feel uncomfortable at first, but with practice, it will feel more natural.

Greg shared that the best thing someone said to him was "Greg, I heard about Staci. I am really sorry. Is there anything I can do to support you specifically?" Short, sweet, and specific.

On another note, consistency matters more than most people realize. Be the friend, family member, or colleague who checks in after thirty days, sixty days, or ninety days. In the early weeks, there is often a flurry of care—meals dropped off, flowers delivered, and messages pouring in. The world rallies when pain feels urgent. But as time stretches on, that energy fades. The texts slow, the casseroles stop, and silence begins to fill the spaces where support once lived. That's when presence becomes its own kind of ministry. Show up after the initial noise quiets. Send a message, make a call, or simply sit beside them in ordinary moments. The gesture doesn't have to be grand. What matters is the steadiness of your care—the quiet reminder that they have not been forgotten, even as the world moves on. *Staci chiming in here: I want to emphasize this. The harder parts come in the quiet after the rush of attention. Calendar check-ins or just sending a funny meme let me know you still care.*

Counselor or not, I don't always get it right. I've said things to Staci and my parents I wish I could take back; the key is to own it and apologize when my head and my mouth aren't aligned. These moments occur more often with Staci than with my parents. Here is one of our text exchanges:

Me:	What time is chemo on Friday?
Staci:	It's today at 1:30.
Me:	Ugh, sorry for not remembering the right day 😢.
Staci:	Please let's not have to apologize to each other about all of this!!

I share this so you know that even as a therapist, I absolutely do *not* get it right 100 percent of the time. Not even close.

And then there's my dad . . .

Yesterday, I completely put my foot in my mouth during a phone call with him. He was listing the side effects of his new immunotherapy—diarrhea, painful achiness, just the whole miserable bingo card. And what did I say? What words came out of my allegedly trained, supposedly therapeutic mouth?

"Dad, you know you don't have to continue treatment if it's affecting your quality of life, right?"

Dead silence. I mean dead silence. You could feel the silence through the phone. Stupid, stupid, stupid thing for me to say.

Would I love to show up the right way every single day? Damn straight I would. Is that realistic? Hell no. I'm human.

And this—these imperfect, cringeworthy, foot-in-mouth moments—is precisely where self-compassion must step in. Not shame. Not guilt. Just a gentle reminder that even the people who *teach* emotional regulation for a living still say the wrong thing, still slip up, and still have to circle back and repair relationship fissures. If anything, these moments have made me more creative about how I communicate and stay connected, especially when words come out the wrong way.

STACI

Nobody knows what to say when someone is going through something devastating, and inevitably, we all say the wrong thing at some point. I've learned to lead with grace because I may be crying about something when someone else is laughing about it, or vice versa. I believe laughter is medicine, and chuckling about cancer, death, or other hard things is absolutely okay. There have certainly been funny moments, like the drawing in the oncologist's waiting room for Halloween that had a bride and groom skeleton and the message "Until death do us part." Like the card that said, "Wishing you a full and speedy recovery." Or the time I had to have an unplanned pap smear, and my partner, Greg, who sat through it, said, "Man, this is taking years off my life."

There have also been moments when something someone said just hit me sideways. For example, I just asked Greg yesterday to stop saying, "I could get hit by a bus tomorrow." It feels diminishing to my experience, and the last thing I need is to worry about Greg dying. When something like this happens, I know that person meant no ill will; they were just being honest or funny. All of this is a constant negotiation of emotions, and I've learned to speak up when I need to protect my head, my heart, or both.

What hasn't been helpful is the people who say they'll come see me, then don't, or those with ulterior motives for checking in. I have no patience or space for those people.

The best response I've received happened just a few weeks ago when I told someone I know from a professional setting. They asked, "What do you want me to know about your diagnosis?" Wow. For me, that was the perfect question.

* * *

As you look for other ways to connect with your people, please consider setting up a CaringBridge site. This free, nonprofit online platform lets individuals and families create a private website to share health updates and connect with loved ones during a health journey. It simplifies communication by eliminating the need to repeatedly update people individually and helps coordinate support by allowing users to post requests for help with things like meals or transportation. It has allowed us to share updates on Staci's cancer journey, organize meal support, and create a community of cheerleaders for this warrior. It has taken the pressure off Greg and all of us in that inner circle.

Journaling Exercise

- What phrases comfort you when you're struggling?

- Which ones feel dismissive or unhelpful?

Boundaries with Family, Friends, and the Person Who Is Ill

During serious illness, boundaries become essential. Well-meaning friends may offer unsolicited advice. Family members might project their own fears. Even the person who is ill may ask for more than you can emotionally or physically give.

Boundaries are self-defined limits that clarify what you will and will not accept in relationships. Communicated through your own choices and behavior, they protect your time, energy, and emotional/physical safety without trying to manage another person. They are forms of self-care and respect that foster healthier interactions and relationships.

Boundaries are not barriers—they are a form of love that protects your energy and preserves relationships. Saying "no" or "not right now" does not mean you don't care; it means you are caring for yourself so you can continue to show up with presence and compassion. This is particularly important if you are serving as someone's caregiver.

Everyone has different values, needs, and sensitivities, so the process of defining personal boundaries can vary from person to person. Your boundaries will also change over the course of your life as you learn more about yourself and what you value.

There are three types of boundaries. They are rigid, porous, and healthy.

Rigid boundaries are unyielding and absolute. Rigid boundaries do a good job of protecting you, but they do so at a cost. They create distance between you and the people in your life, potentially harming your relationships. If you have a fear of vulnerability or a history of relationships in which you were taken advantage of, you may be more likely to adopt rigid boundaries.

A rigid boundary often sounds like "my way or the highway." It can come across as detached or cold, leaving little room for flexibility. For example, your mother asks you to meet her for lunch at a deli you dislike. You refuse and offer no alternative, effectively shutting down the interaction. Or consider a partner who asks to talk after a disagreement. Rather than expressing a need for space, you abruptly announce, "I'm done with this conversation" and walk away, making it clear there is no opportunity to reconnect or clarify.

In caregiving, a rigid boundary might look like refusing all offers of help because you believe no one can do it "right." When your sibling offers to take your dad to an appointment, you immediately decline without discussion, not because it won't work but because you're unwilling to share the responsibility. This protects you from discomfort in the moment, but it also increases your burden and keeps others at arm's length.

Porous boundaries fall at the other end of the spectrum. They are weak and easily breached. This type of boundary can show up as oversharing information with others and having a difficult time saying "no." People who are afraid of rejection or emotionally entangled with others are more likely to have porous boundaries. Most people pleasers have porous boundaries.

A porous boundary sounds like this: frequently saying "yes" to requests you don't want to do, even when it compromises your own well-being or desires. You might say "yes" out of guilt or fear of rejection, telling yourself, *As long as everyone else is happy, I'm happy.* But are you?

Porous boundaries can also look like telling a new coworker deeply personal details about your family or relationship before trust has been established. Or immediately absorbing someone else's crisis—dropping your plans, rearranging your schedule, and prioritizing their needs over your own without being asked. In caregiving, it might show up as taking on every task because you feel guilty asking siblings for help or letting a loved one's frustration or disappointment dictate your choices.

Healthy boundaries fall somewhere between rigid and porous. This is a healthy boundary (flexible + respectful): "I'd love to see you. That deli doesn't work for me, though. How about the café on Peachtree or the Thai place near you? If neither works, let's pick another place."

Why it's healthy: It states a need ("That deli doesn't work for me"), keeps the connection ("I'd love to see you"), and offers viable alternatives. Your boundary is about what you will do—"I'll do X, but I won't do Y to protect my time, energy, and well-being."

Greg talked about the boundaries he had to set when Staci first started chemotherapy with Cisplatin. It made her sick and immunocompromised. "I had to keep people from visiting too long to preserve her energy and protect her health." While asking people to leave was difficult, this was Greg's way of keeping Staci safe. He also shared a boundary he set for Leadership Atlanta. He chose not to go to this year's opening retreat. "I noticed people treating me like a sad puppy, like they expect me to unburden myself with them. I want to bring up Staci's cancer on my terms."

Here are some additional examples for context:

- **Time:** "I can talk until 8 p.m. After that, I need to rest. If we're not done, let's schedule a call tomorrow when I am rested."
- **Work hours:** "I don't check email after 7 p.m. I'll respond in the morning."
- **Topic:** "I'm not up for discussing my treatment today. We can talk about it on Friday, but today, let's keep it light."

Examples for specific groups:

- **With friends:** "I appreciate your concern, but I'm not ready to share details right now."
- **With family:** "I need a break from caregiving this weekend. Can we arrange a schedule so we share the load?"
- **With the person who is ill:** "I love you, and I want to be here. I also need a little time each day to recharge."

Setting boundaries is one part of caring for both yourself and others. Boundaries clarify what you can offer without resentment or exhaustion. But once you've made space for your own well-being, the next question often becomes: *How can I still show up for the people I love in meaningful ways?*

Support doesn't always mean doing everything; it means knowing what kind of helper you are and where your presence matters most. In fact, research and lived experience show that the quality of support matters more than the quantity.

That's why I love the framework published by National Public Radio in an article titled "Appointment buddy or meal planner? 4 ways to support a friend with cancer."[13] While written for friends of cancer patients, the guidance applies to any caregiving or anticipatory grief situation.

What Kind of Helper Are You?

Staci sent me the article I referenced above. The author, Marielle Segarra, says, "There are four specific roles that friends and family members can play for a loved one with cancer. They each meet a critical need that cancer patients often have."[14] Those roles include doctor appointment buddy, procedure pal/patient advocate, post-surgery/post-treatment companion, and household helper/meal planner. Here is how those roles were defined:

1. **Doctor appointment buddy:** This is good for you if "you're organized, detail-oriented, and comfortable in medical environments."[15] This person prepares questions and takes notes during doctor's appointments, since the information is too much for one person to absorb.

    Staci: Early on, there was so much information coming at us, and we had to go back to the same building a gazillion times. It was so helpful to have Tim there with Greg and me at "chemo camp." We made a rule: I was not going to go to that building alone.

2. **Procedure pal/patient advocate:** "You're the kind of person who is comfortable with physical touch, sitting in silence, praying, or even bringing your best comedy routine (depending on the person's mood). You should also be willing to advocate for your loved one if needed."[16] If you are comfortable speaking up or questioning a medical decision, this may be the spot for you.

Tim is great at this; he's especially adept at cracking jokes to lighten the mood.

Staci: At first, chemo was really rough, and I just wanted my closest people there. But now that I am past the heavy chemo, it has become a great way to catch up with friends. You have these dedicated hours together to laugh, cry, and create new memories. I go every three weeks for chemo, and now I think about who would be fun to go with.

3. **Post-surgery/post-treatment companion:** You can do this if "you have a strong stomach (you might see blood, burns, or healing incisions), and if you're able to be mentally strong despite seeing your loved one at a low point."[17] Not everyone can do this role. It's tough.

   Staci: This was Amy for me. She wanted to be there for the hardest stuff, and she was so good at it. She was there for my treatment plan, my first four chemo sessions, and my port implantation. This amazing human walked into my office one day in Florida and said, "I want your job someday." That began the most incredible friendship. Amy has put up with more of my shenanigans than anyone. And we've had the best adventures. We have lived together and worked together, and through it all, we have remained best friends.

4. **Household helper/meal planner:** This is for you if "you're good at organizing and planning and willing to take initiative."[18] The person in this role helps with meal trains, grocery shopping, and cleaning schedules

for living spaces. These tasks will significantly reduce the patient's workload.

Staci: This was for Frances and Meagan. Meagan set up a meal train for us, and it was the most helpful thing ever. It took the load off of deciding what to cook and the chore of cooking when I didn't want to. Our village really showed up in this way, and I was so sad when it ended—haha! Frances sent us cookbooks and meal storage containers and would have been there every week to meal prep had she not ended up in the ER a week after my diagnosis with her husband. That is a whole different story, but it has been so hard for Frances and me. Our friendship seems so much stronger, even though we are both navigating life-changing crises and chaos.

The NPR framework offers a way to think about how support might look on paper—defined, organized, and intentional. But real life rarely unfolds that neatly. Illness has a way of exposing the difference between what people *intend* to offer and what they can *actually* do. It reveals the quiet truths about connection—who shows up, who pulls away, and who surprises you altogether.

For Staci, those lessons became deeply personal.

STACI

My relationships shifted in ways I couldn't have predicted after my diagnosis. I've been stunned by the outpouring of love and support. People I haven't spoken with in years reached out, reminding me of the quiet power of kindness and how connection can reappear when you need it most. At the same time, I couldn't care less about the folks who seem to feel a performative "need" to check in. There is a person in my life who checked in a lot in the beginning. We had just had this weird, unresolved experience, so there was unspoken tension for me. They offered help, but I did not feel like it was authentic. I finally stopped responding. My focus is on my people and my family—they know who they are—and on the ones who show up with steadiness rather than spectacle.

There have been some powerful moments that will be core memories for me, like the day I got my port and had chemo the same day. I had made it through surgery, and the surgeon even told Greg that I was the most cheerful patient he had ever met. But that mask fell off quickly when fear set in. I had no experience with a port, and I was scared of what it would feel like when they inserted it. (A port is a semi-permanent device placed in your chest for direct access to your bloodstream for treatment. It sits right under your skin, and the needle goes directly into it during treatment.)

Amy knew exactly what to do. She walked over to my bed, took my hand, looked me in the eyes, and said, "You've got this. You can do this." Then she went and got me some mac and cheese because I hadn't eaten all day and stayed up with me gabbing until we finally got to go home at 5:30 in the morning.

I will never forget Liz being in the ER with me. I have no clue how she got there, but she was so brave and calm, never flinching. She went with me to my room and held space for everything I was feeling. The next day, I had hand-drawn pictures from Liz and Jack's adorable kids, some dry shampoo, and homemade soup for dinner.

Oh, yeah, you need to meet Liz! Liz and I met through a mentor/mentee program. Neither of us was very sure why we were paired together. Our careers were in such different arenas. Yet something clicked when we met the first time—maybe because I asked her about her sex life. The sex educator in me just couldn't help it! Our friendship quickly evolved, and Greg and I met her partner, Jack, the night he proposed. Greg preached at their wedding, and we still gather for a Sunday supper ritual born in COVID that has now lasted for five years.

I needed a place to be after chemo, and Meagan, Tim, and Jack made that happen. On top of being a best friend, an amazing therapist, and an awesome dog mom, Meagan also has a keen eye for decorating. She went with me to look for furniture, and we found the perfect pieces. Tim rented a U-Haul. Tim, Jack, and Greg moved everything in one day. Then Meagan took the reins and made the most beautiful gallery wall with all our art. Every time I sit in that space that now feels like my very own cave, I think of that day and my people who created a safe, warm space for me.

The relationships that have become most important are the ones that combine presence, practicality, and respect for boundaries. And meaning has shown up in my relationships. There's been real healing between Greg and Amy, which has brought me so much peace. They both had their own reasons for their feelings about the other, but all that has faded away. My mom insists on a morning FaceTime call that gives me a rhythm of comfort and joy. My dearest college friend, Brett, immediately made himself the arbiter of honesty and my source of "special" healing aids. I hear more often from my sisters-in-law. People from all parts of my life have signed up to be a real part of this experience. And you know what? I'm not mad or disappointed in anyone I haven't heard from. The reality is that you can't walk in someone else's shoes, so you never know what they're holding or juggling.

Things have been hard too. One of our closest friends had a life-altering medical event exactly one week after I went to the ER. His wife, Frances, and I would have been ALL IN IT for each other if we hadn't been knee-deep in our own crises. That has sucked. And for my precious parents, this has been gut-wrenching. Every time we have to deliver hard news, it rips a piece of my heart out.

I was pleasantly surprised by a handful of people who showed up with exactly what I needed: quiet reliability, thoughtful texts, rides, meals, and humor when the air got heavy. Their consistency mattered more than perfect words. On the harder side, I'm still sorting through what to do about my biological mom. Old anger and fresh grief sit side by side there, and I'm taking my time and protecting my head and heart while I decide what connection, if any, is healthy for me.

In the end, the "why" behind who matters most is simple: They made space for my reality, honored my boundaries, brought light without minimizing the dark, could laugh at all the things, and stood still with me in uncertainty. These are the people who stepped up and never left.

Journaling Exercise

Spot the Pattern

- In the last week, when did I say "yes" but mean "no"? What was I afraid would happen if I declined?

- What was the earliest moment I noticed discomfort in that situation?

Body and Emotional Cues

- Where in my body do I feel "boundary pressure" (jaw, chest, stomach)? What's the first sensation?

- Which emotions tend to signal I need a boundary (resentment, dread, overwhelm, irritation)?

Values, Limits, and Consent

- Which value is often violated or ignored (respect, rest, honesty, fairness, privacy) when someone crosses my boundary?

- Complete the sentence: "I am willing to ____________; I am **not** willing to ____________."

Fear and Stories

- What story keeps me from setting a boundary (e.g., "They'll leave," "I'm selfish," "Conflict is dangerous")?

Debrief After Setting a Boundary

- How do I self-soothe after setting a boundary (breathing, walking, listening to music, calling a friend)?

- Did the outcome align with my values, even if it felt uncomfortable?

Progress Tracking (Weekly)

- Times I set a boundary: ___ Times I wish I had: ___
- Average resentment or other emotion I felt (use a scale of 0–10) **before** vs. **after** boundary work.

Shifts in Roles

Illness can change the shape of relationships overnight. Friends may become caregivers. Children may find themselves making decisions for their parents, like I did when my dad underwent kidney surgery. Siblings may take on new responsibilities. These role changes often carry their own grief—loss of the relationship as it once was.

Acknowledging the shift is the first step. You may not be able to return to the old dynamic, but you can still honor it. For example, a daughter caring for her father might say: "I'll always be your child, even as I help with these decisions. That part of us doesn't change."

Parenting a Parent: When Love Requires Decisions

Bentina is a dear friend I met through Leadership Atlanta. She is another remarkable leader, serving as the current president and CEO of Southern Linc and Southern Telecom, Inc., subsidiaries of the Southern Company. Bentina is intelligent, compassionate, and charismatic and has a true passion for helping nonprofits in her not-so-spare time. You should google her—she is that impressive. Despite all her responsibilities, she makes time for her people, and I love that I get to be part of that tribe.

For a long time, Bentina's father believed he had a back problem. After years of jumping out of helicopters as a soldier, he thought pain was the natural cost of a hard life. When he finally underwent back surgery and became septic, something shifted for Bentina—not only because of the surgery but because her brother had died quickly and unexpectedly from sepsis just six months earlier. Sitting in that hospital room, still raw from her brother's death, was the first time she allowed herself to think, *I could lose my dad too.*

When her father was diagnosed with ALS roughly six months later, Bentina didn't fully understand what it meant. She only knew this: They were going to lose him slowly, and it was going to hurt.

The early months were filled with trying to understand what ALS was, how it would progress, and what it would take from him. At first, the losses were subtle. Then they weren't.

One of the first battles was over driving. Her father was stubborn, proud, and fiercely independent. Bentina was terrified. She worried he would hurt himself—or someone else. They argued vehemently. It was the first time she realized their roles had shifted. She was no longer only his daughter. She was becoming his parent.

She hated it.

He hated it more.

Parenting a parent is a special kind of hell—necessary, intimate, and profoundly unnatural.

As the disease progressed, milestones arrived whether the family was ready or not. The walker became a wheelchair. They'd tried to keep him walking for as long as possible, knowing that once he sat in the chair, he would never walk again. The finality of that moment took her breath away.

Then came the conversation about a feeding tube.

The medical team explained that the procedure needed to happen while his body could still withstand surgery. If he waited too long, the option would disappear. But her father said no.

Bentina remembers sitting down with him to speak on behalf of the family. She asked if he understood that if he lost the ability to swallow, he would die.

"Yes," he said. "I understand. If I can't swallow, I don't want to live."

Hearing him say it hurt. Still, she told him it was okay and that she would explain it to everyone else. Loving him meant honoring his decision—even when it terrified her.

As time passed, the care became more intimate.

She remembers having to change him after he soiled himself. She could see the humiliation on his face. She smiled and told him, "You did it for me first," then kissed him, hoping it helped. She wasn't sure if it did. She couldn't imagine what it felt like to have her children wiping her body when it no longer worked the way it once did.

For a long time, her father was depressed. He asked why God was keeping him alive. Why had he become a burden? She didn't have any answers.

And then, one day, something shifted.

He stopped asking why. He said it was okay—that he was at peace. Bentina could feel it—an unmistakable serenity settling into the room.

Not long after that, she cried in front of him. Her mother never wanted them to do that, but she couldn't stop herself. When he asked why, she told him the truth.

"Because you're dying."

He looked at her and said, "Squeak, we're all dying. Every day. You just know what will kill me."

His seventy-ninth birthday came five months before he died. He called her, thrilled.

"I made it," he said. "I made it to seventy-nine."

She laughed with him. "Happy birthday, Poppi."

When she hung up the phone, she sobbed.

That moment—joy braided tightly with grief—marks the kind of threshold anticipatory grief so often creates. Nothing had ended yet, but everything had already changed. Love was still present. Time was not.

Bentina's story carries us through the long arc of illness and caregiving. It shows us what happens when uncertainty gives way to responsibility, when vigilance becomes care, and when love demands decisions no child ever expects to make.

Not every story of anticipatory grief looks like this. Some unfold quietly, before diagnosis. Some begin not with illness but with noticing—small changes, subtle shifts, moments that don't yet have names.

That's where my story begins.

I've noticed a shift in my relationships with my parents over the last two to three years. While three of them have shown minimal cognitive decline, they are slowing down. My dad has been battling bladder cancer and, at the same time, caring for my stepmother, who has Alzheimer's. During one visit, we had to have "the conversation," or discuss, as I like to call it, "the business of family." That becomes particularly true when it comes to finances and long-term care. My dad and stepmom have both done an exceptional job preparing for retirement and death. A trust exists, and it is no surprise that I am the executor. That piece is heavy by itself.

What was heavier was the conversation Tim and I had with my dad about what would happen if he died first. That was not a fun conversation, but it was an important one. What was the care plan? Did his wife, Becky, want to be at home? Had they looked at any long-term care facilities? My dad could have reacted in many ways, including being angry. I wondered about that on the flight back to Atlanta.

On Monday, after we left, my dad shared an article from Axios titled "Power of Now." In the article, Jim VandeHei wrote about Mike Allen, "[He's] the hardest working person I've ever met, never hesitates to move instantly on, well, anything he deems important."[19]

One specific callout resonated with me. It read, "If he's going to connect with someone, he does it now. Apologize? Now. You wanna get lunch? How's tomorrow? Start a new health habit? On it!"[20]

So what does this look like in practice? Here are three of Allen's seven bullet points that resonate with me:[21]

1. "If something is important, do it today. Why wait until Monday to start eating healthier (one last binge!) or next weekend to call your parents or next month to start running again? Every hour you wait increases the chance you'll simply blow it off . . . again.
2. If you need to have a tough conversation with a friend, family member, or colleague, do it now. This is where everyone drags their feet too long, too often. The problem spreads and deepens. You prolong your anxiety about the tough talk. Every minute you dither is another minute of pain and another minute that person is not spending fixing their issue—or solving yours.
3. It can save your life. If you notice a blemish, or know you should get a test or exam, putting it off can be fatal. We know our bodies; we're creatures of habit. And if you suddenly feel funny or notice something worrisome, act on it if you're lucky enough to have care available. Sadly, just about every one of us has a loved one who regrets waiting."

My dad was not upset by our conversation and did understand the urgency. Delivering it via an article is just his style. On our last trip to visit, we ended up putting my stepmother on a waiting list for a memory care center, and I am immensely relieved by that development. I am really good at these challenging conversations. It is my superpower. You can be too with a bit of practice.

Journaling Exercise

- How has your role changed in this relationship? What do you miss about how it used to be?

- What role do you need to take on?

- What is left unsaid between you and your loved one?

Chapter 6

THE BODY REMEMBERS

I will never forget the morning when my body told the truth before my mind was willing to catch up. I was sitting in my car on the street beside my house, hands wrapped around the steering wheel, unable to make myself walk inside. Nothing dramatic happened that day, no new diagnosis, no crisis. But my chest felt tight, my stomach churned, and a wave of exhaustion rolled through me so heavy it felt suffocating.

I kept telling myself, *You're fine. Just push through. You don't have time for this.*

But my body disagreed.

It was only later, with some distance and my therapist's gentle nudge, that I recognized what was happening: My nervous system was trying to get my attention. Weeks of holding Staci's illness, my family obligations, my clients, and the quiet fears I refused to name had finally overflowed. My body remembered the stress I kept trying to outthink.

That moment became a turning point for me—a reminder that grief isn't just emotional. It is physical and cellular, affecting your whole body. And if you ignore the early signs, your body and mind will eventually insist you listen.

So this is your reminder: Grief shows up in both your body and your mind. If you need a refresher, revisit Chapter 3.

So far, we have defined anticipatory grief, explored its manifestations, and examined its emotional, mental, and physical effects. Now, we will focus specifically on mental health—and how to recognize when it's essential to seek additional support. I am going to try to keep this as straightforward and nonacademic as I can. Navigating the mental health system can be daunting, so I believe straight talk is the best approach.

What Do We Mean by Mental Health?

Mental health refers to your emotional, psychological, social, and spiritual well-being. It shapes how you manage stress, relate to others, and make decisions. It also changes over time in response to life's demands. When those demands begin to exceed your available resources, your capacity to cope and function day to day can falter.

For example, let's talk about Eric—caring for his mother, who has a chronic illness, while juggling a demanding job and pretending he can survive on protein bars and three hours of sleep. His day starts at 5:30 a.m. because his mom needs help getting situated before he heads into the office. On the drive to work, he's already mentally cataloging: *Did I reschedule her cardiology appointment? Did I order more meds? Why did I agree to host the team meeting today?* At lunchtime, he's fielding texts from his mom's home health nurse, the pharmacy, and his boss—none of whom seem to coordinate their crises with one another.

By late afternoon, he's running on fumes. He tries to answer a simple email but stares at the screen as if it's written in ancient Sanskrit. On the way home, he has a minor meltdown in the Kroger parking lot because he can't remember whether he was supposed to buy whole milk, almond milk, or oat milk. (Spoiler: It was oat milk. His mom is very committed to her digestive peace.)

And when he finally sits down for the night—exhausted, overstretched, and emotionally frayed—Eric wonders why he feels so forgetful, irritable, and on edge. The truth? He isn't failing. His system is simply operating far beyond capacity. He's in survival mode, pulling from a well that's been dry for a long time.

Grief works the same way. When someone is carrying the weight of an impending loss, their emotional bandwidth narrows dramatically. They may find themselves crying in their car after holding it together all day, forgetting important appointments, or moving through the world like everything is happening two seconds too fast. Even the routine stuff—paying bills, replying to messages, deciding what to cook for dinner—can suddenly feel impossible.

This isn't a lack of resilience. It's the natural consequence of doing enormous emotional labor while trying to keep life moving forward.

When we look at it through this lens, it becomes clear that these struggles aren't signs of weakness—they're human responses to overwhelming circumstances. And because these experiences are so universal, we must talk about them impacting our mental health openly rather than treating them as something rare or shameful.

Because mental health touches so many of us, I work hard to normalize it as "just health." Consider a few quick facts you've likely seen: Many adults will experience a mental health condition at some point, and only about half receive treatment.

Given how common this is, we need everyday language that makes mental health accessible. With loved ones—or with yourself—try: "How are you, really?" "Tell me how you're feeling." "You seem down—how can I support you?" Normalize, normalize, normalize.

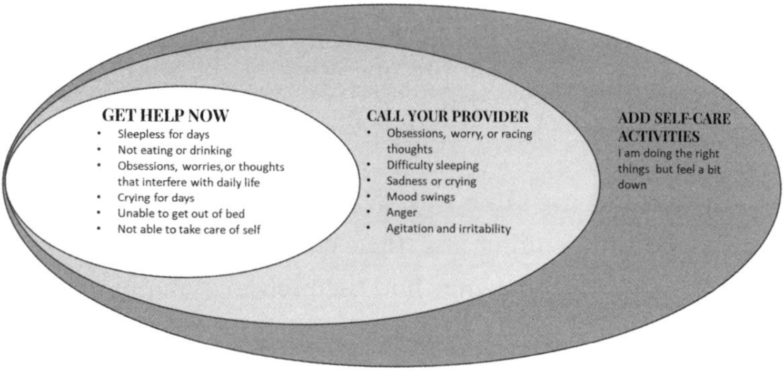

Let me give you some quick stats:[22]

- Twenty percent of, or one in five, adults in the United States will experience mental illness this year alone. Only 50 percent get treatment.
- Forty-six percent of adults in the United States will meet the criteria for a diagnosable mental health condition sometime in their life.
- Fifty percent of mental health conditions appear before the age of fourteen and 75 percent by the age of twenty-four.

It isn't always easy to distinguish expected ups and downs from signs of a mental health condition. Watch for persistent mood changes; ongoing fear, worry, or panic that's hard to turn off; pulling back from friends, family, or activities you usually enjoy; changes in sleep, appetite, energy, or concentration that last for weeks; using alcohol or substances to cope; and thoughts of hopelessness, self-harm, or suicide. These symptoms matter not only in themselves but in how they affect your life. A mental health disorder can interfere with your ability to:[23]

- Maintain relationships.
- Manage social situations.
- Perform at work or school.
- Participate in typical daily activities.
- Learn at a level expected for your age and intelligence.

Grief can complicate this picture because intense grief often mimics depression or anxiety—restlessness, tearfulness, brain fog, disrupted sleep. Two anchors help clinicians sort it out: time (are symptoms easing, staying flat, or worsening?) and impairment and safety (is daily functioning impaired, and are there thoughts of self-harm?). If symptoms persist, escalate, or significantly impact your life, it's time for a professional evaluation—regardless of the cause.

Think of getting a diagnosis for a mental health condition as a way of understanding what's going on—not as a judgment and definitely not as a life sentence. Clinicians use a book called the *Diagnostic and Statistical Manual of Mental Disorders (DSM)*, which outlines the criteria for hundreds of conditions like anxiety, depression, eating disorders, PTSD, and schizophrenia.

But in real life, it looks less like checking boxes and more like listening for patterns:

- Someone might come in saying, "I can't sleep anymore, I'm crying on the way to work, and I feel like I'm failing at everything." A clinician gently explores when it started, how long it's been happening, and how it's affecting daily life.
- Another person might describe panic attacks that feel like heart attacks. A clinician considers the frequency, the triggers, and whether physical causes have been ruled out.
- Someone experiencing grief may appear fine to others, but a clinician notices signs of prolonged sadness, withdrawal, or exhaustion that point to depression layered on top of grief.

The goal isn't to put you into a category—it's to understand you well enough to help.

Great. So now what?

Once a diagnosis (or working hypothesis) is made, it becomes a road map. It helps guide what kind of therapy might work best, whether medication could help, and whether your general practitioner should check out some symptoms. It's like saying, "Okay, now we know what we're dealing with. Here's what we can do about it."

Who Can Diagnose?

Licensed mental health professionals—psychiatrists, psychologists, counselors, and clinical social workers—are trained to assess, diagnose, and treat.

For many people, the first stop is their **primary care clinician**. They can ensure that your symptoms aren't being caused by a physical ailment and connect you with a mental health professional. Or they may also start you on an antidepressant or other medication based on a quick office assessment if you are in immediate distress or can't access a specialist quickly.

The tricky part is that mental health symptoms often look like everyday life stress: Is your friend withdrawing because they're "busy" or because they're overwhelmed? Are you exhausted because you're working too much or because grief has pulled the plug on your emotional energy?

That is why it's essential to know who to go to for help—and what kind of training they have.

Psychiatrists are medical doctors who can evaluate medical factors (thyroid issues, pain, insomnia, hormones) and prescribe medications. Some also do therapy.

General practitioners now write many mental health prescriptions, especially when someone is in crisis or can't access a specialist. This is one more reminder that mental health is just health.

Psychologists conduct therapy and psychological testing. They often specialize in specific approaches like cognitive behavioral therapy, eye movement desensitization and reprocessing, or health psychology.

Licensed professional counselors (LPCs), licensed clinical social workers (LCSWs), and **licensed marriage and family therapists (LMFTs)** provide counseling, diagnose, coordinate care, and connect clients with real-world support and tools.

Now, let me step onto my soapbox for a moment.

Almost anyone can use the term *therapist*—me included. It's not a legally protected title. And this matters.

When someone is scared, overwhelmed, or reaching out for help for the first time, they're often at their most vulnerable. They deserve to know they're sitting across from someone with real training, ethical accountability, and supervision—not someone who took an online course and bought a business card.

Without clear protections around the title, people can unknowingly place their trust in someone who isn't equipped to handle complex trauma, crisis, or grief.

So here's the difference:

- Psychiatrists hold a medical degree (MD).
- Psychologists earned a doctoral degree (PhD or PsyD).
- LPCs, LMFTs, and LCSWs all hold master's degrees and completed more than two thousand supervised clinical hours before full licensure.

These titles are legally protected. That means the person using them has passed exams, has completed extensive training, and follows strict ethical and legal standards. That's why checking credentials matters—you deserve safe, qualified care.

Now that I've stepped off my soapbox . . . let's talk about what happens next. And that starts with finding a provider that makes sense for you.

How Do You Find a Provider?

To get started, identify a provider through your insurance directory (although some of the best do not accept insurance), a primary care referral, or reputable listings such as state licensure boards, hospital systems, trusted community organizations, or sites like Psychology Today. A more robust list will be available in the back of this book. Prepare for the initial call by jotting down your top concerns and when they started. Be prepared to talk about your sleep, appetite, energy, and concentration for the last two weeks. Make sure you have a list of all medications and supplements and note any family history of mental health or substance use, even if it is undiagnosed.

If you are considering counseling, the professional should offer a free fifteen- to twenty-minute initial consultation so you can determine whether they are the right fit for you or a loved one.

It can be scary to interview a mental health provider, but it is a crucial part of the process. You need to believe that you can grow to trust your provider and build rapport. Here are my suggested questions to ask:

- Are you licensed to practice in my state?
- How long have you been practicing in the mental health space?
- What are your specialties?
- What are my options—therapy types, self-care strategies, medication—and what are the pros/cons of each?
- How will we measure progress, and when will we adjust the plan?
- How often will we meet?
- What do I do between sessions?
- Have you worked with clients who have similar experiences to mine?
- In your experience, how long will it take me to feel better?

At its core, this process is simply a way of shining a light on what you've been carrying—often alone, often for far too long. It's not about labeling you or defining your future; it's about giving language to describe your experience and symptoms so you can finally get the support you deserve.

Once you find a provider who feels like a good fit, the next step is scheduling an initial intake session. This first appointment typically lasts about an hour and serves as the starting point for understanding your needs.

An initial evaluation usually covers your story and timeline—when symptoms began, how they've evolved, and what has happened in your life before and during your grief experience. They may ask what worsens or relieves your symptoms and wish to understand the context of your grief or other life stressors—followed by conducting a check on sleep, appetite, energy, focus, work or school performance, and relationships. Clinicians assess safety and substance use, complete a brief mental status exam (mood, thought patterns, orientation, insight), and outline a plan that might include education, therapy, lifestyle changes, and, when appropriate, medication or lab work.

While I've talked about generalities here, let me elaborate on how I approach an initial intake assessment. For me, the most crucial part of this first session is building trust. If you can't trust your counselor, social worker, psychologist, or psychiatrist, the relationship simply won't work—no matter how many degrees they have hanging on their wall.

Once we begin, I ask questions that help me get a fuller picture of who my client is and what brought them in. At the top of the session, I'll ask things like:

- When you called to make an appointment, what was going on?
- What do you want to get out of this experience? What are your expectations or goals?
- Have you seen a counselor before? What was that experience like? What worked and what didn't?

From there, I transition to questions about their mental health history as well as their family's—diagnosed or not. Honestly, I often get more clarity when I ask about *undiagnosed* mental health conditions. Those answers sound like, "I'm pretty sure my mom is anxious," or "My dad struggled with depression." That information matters because it helps me understand what may be happening in their body and mind on a day-to-day basis.

Next, I want to get a sense of how they think. I typically ask something like, "How do you approach problem-solving?" then follow up with how that plays out in both their personal and professional lives. After that, we go deeper into family history, work, and support systems. Some questions sound like:

- Who do you count on in your life? Tell me about the important relationships—give me names, roles, and why those people matter.
- What was it like growing up in your home? How did your family handle conflict?
- Tell me about your work. How do you feel about what you do?

Then, we move into lifestyle and self-care habits because, as unglamorous as it sounds, these things matter. I ask about appetite and the kinds of foods they eat. What you eat and drink can impact your mood, so I need a general sense of their baseline. For example, did you know dehydration can exacerbate anxiety? I'm not suggesting anyone needs to chug a gallon of water a day, but I *am* suggesting that four Diet Cokes do not count as hydration, as one of my clients wants to believe.

From there, I cover sleep: bedtime, wake time, hours, and overall quality. Sleep can dramatically affect mood. Poor or inadequate sleep can lead to irritability and stress, while healthy sleep can enhance emotional well-being. Chronic insomnia may even increase the risk of developing a mood disorder like anxiety or depression. In one major study of ten thousand adults, people with insomnia were five times more likely to develop depression. The same study showed people with insomnia were twenty times more likely to develop panic disorder.[24]

After sleep, I ask about exercise. What do you enjoy doing? And how often are you exercising? Exercising regularly can improve symptoms of mild to moderate depression as well as anxiety and psychological distress.[25]

When I started digging into the research, one theme kept popping up: *Moving your body matters.* And not in an "I run marathons" way. I'm talking about the normal people stuff—walking the dog around the block, doing a YouTube Pilates video in your living room, lifting a couple of dumbbells that have been collecting dust since 2018, or rolling out a yoga mat because your therapist said it might help (and I would be that therapist).

Across study after study, people who were even a little bit active—just doing the things that felt doable—saw real improvements in their mood. The walkers, the lifters, the yogis, the Pilates crew . . . all of them reported feeling less weighed down by symptoms of mild to moderate depression. Yoga and other mind–body exercises stood out for easing anxiety, as if whispering to the nervous system, "Let's take it down a notch." Meanwhile, resistance training was the quiet MVP for lifting depressive symptoms.

Toward the end of the intake, I ask my favorite question: What did I not ask you that you think is important for me to know? It opens the door for anything I may have missed—because sometimes the most crucial detail doesn't surface until the very end of the session.

After that, I ask if they have any questions for me. And before outlining the next steps, I ask directly: Do you think you'll be comfortable working with me? It's okay if the answer is no. I'm happy to help you find someone who's a better fit.

If they are comfortable, we schedule the next appointment and begin setting treatment goals during the following session. This is usually when people start to wonder what therapy will actually *look* like—what happens in the room, how I approach their concerns, and what tools I might use. Every mental health professional takes a different approach to therapy sessions. There are literally dozens of approaches, from art therapy to written exposure therapy.[26]

What I am going to highlight are four of the most commonly used approaches. It does not mean these are right for you. There are many different approaches to therapy, and each one offers something unique depending on your needs. **Cognitive behavioral therapy (CBT)** is a structured, short-term approach that helps people identify and change unhelpful thought patterns and behaviors—making it especially effective for anxiety and depression. **Psychodynamic therapy**, on the other hand, looks beneath the surface. It explores, often through open-ended talk therapy, how unconscious patterns and past experiences shape the way you think, feel, and relate to others today. For those who experience intense emotions or big swings in moods, **dialectical behavior therapy (DBT)** blends elements of CBT with skills in mindfulness, distress tolerance, emotional regulation, and healthier communication. And then there's **humanistic therapy**, which centers on your capacity for growth, emphasizing self-discovery, personal meaning, and the belief that you already hold the potential to move toward your most authentic life. Together, these approaches offer a range of healing pathways that can resonate with you and your story.

And now a word on medication. Of the types of professionals I have outlined in this chapter, only physicians and psychiatrists can prescribe medication. Research shows that some symptoms of mental illness come from chemical imbalances in a person's brain. Medication works on these imbalances to reduce your symptoms or, in some cases, relieve them entirely. It may take some trial and error until you find a medication that makes sense for you, so it is essential to be honest with your physician about any improvements and side effects.

Here's my personal opinion on medication: Would you take insulin for diabetes? A statin for high cholesterol? Aspirin for a headache? If the answer is yes, then the same logic applies to medication for mental health conditions. It's no different. As I will describe in more detail shortly, medication has been life-changing for me personally. I've also had the privilege of watching clients experience significant, sometimes dramatic improvement when they combine counseling with medication. In fact, this combination is the fastest way to reduce symptoms and find relief.

When you know who to turn to and what to expect, the process becomes far less intimidating and far more empowering.

Understanding your mental health is an act of care, clarity, and courage. And once you have that foundation, you can begin the real work of healing, growing, and finding your way forward just like Staci and I have.

STACI

Grief isn't just a feeling; it's a full-body event. My body tells the story even when my words are slow to catch up. Lately, the most visible sign is tears—more of them, more often. Crying has become a pressure valve, my nervous system's way of releasing what my mind can't neatly file away. I used to apologize for it. Now, I try to let it happen and notice how, afterward, my shoulders drop a half inch and my breath loosens, evidence that my body is doing its best to help me survive what hurts.

There's also a new kind of quiet inside me. Sometimes, it feels calm; sometimes, it edges into loneliness. It's the stillness that comes after a wave, when everything is tender and a little too loud. I am learning to name that loneliness without making it mean something is wrong with me. It's a companion to loss, not a personal failing.

In my first therapy session after I got home from the hospital, my therapist asked me if I wanted to live. I was caught off guard by the question, but my instinct was to say, "Yes, I want to live." She told me I needed to tell my body that as often as possible because I may have heard other messages in my lifetime, and I needed to build new neural pathways. These new pathways are fragile and need to be nurtured. That is work.

So that means . . . counseling is the backbone of my mental health care. Having a place to speak the unvarnished truth with a therapist who is willing to push traditional boundaries, to say the thing out loud and let it exist, keeps me from carrying it alone. Therapy helps me separate the story my fear tells from what is actually happening in my body right now. And my therapy is evolving every session. I feel past the acuteness of my diagnosis and can weave back in some of the work we were doing before April 2025. I feel like I am mostly approaching this with a healthy perspective by caring for my mental health and not pretending that I am fine. I say "mostly" because there are days when I catch myself saying, "Nothing has changed in my life except cancer." Girl, EVERYTHING has changed!

I'm also listening to my body with more respect than ever. Sometimes, that looks like honoring what it needs: rest, gentler days, fewer demands. Sometimes, it looks like giving it what it wants: a glass of champagne or a soda, a trashy TV show, a mind-numbing game—because nourishment doesn't have to be "earned." I'm done negotiating with my limits; they're not the enemy—they're information.

I make room for escape that soothes rather than numbs. Reading is one of those doors I can walk through when the edges are too sharp. A chapter becomes a soft place for my mind to land, far enough from the medical words to breathe, close enough to return when I'm ready. I've gotten books from friends about managing cancer, but those are just not where my mind wants to spend its energy right now.

Meditation is often suggested by people, but meditation always starts with breath cues, and that throws me off from the start. When every practice begins with "focus on your breath," I want to scream, "That is the problem!" So I've found other pathways: Nature sounds can settle me without demanding attention from the very system that feels threatened. A low river, distant birds, wind through leaves—these are the rhythms I borrow when I need to steady myself.

I'm guarding my mind with a lot of quiet input, like fewer tabs open (well, that's the goal), more intentional pauses. Quiet lowers the static so I can hear the small signals: I'm tired, I'm overloaded, I need a walk, I should call someone I love.

Through it all runs a simple rule: Feel what I'm feeling and protect the space around myself. Cry when the tears come. Ask for help before the cliff. Choose the tools that actually comfort my body, not the ones that look good on paper. Grief has taken up residence in my muscles, my breath, and my routines, so my care has to live there too.

*   *   *

Counseling was normalized for me from an incredibly young age. My mom was a nurse, and she believed that sometimes you needed professional support to sort things out and build coping skills to feel better. I went to counseling for the first time in my early teens to work through some specific issues related to my dad. Divorce is hard, especially when your parents are in two different states. My mom has also battled depression throughout her life, and she modeled the right behavior by getting help. I am eternally grateful that I grew up in an environment where mental health support was accepted.

I was diagnosed with anxiety in 2017 by my internal medicine physician, who included a screening as part of my annual wellness exam. After much discussion, we decided I needed to start medication, as my symptoms were not resolving with regular self-care efforts. What I appreciated most about Dr.

Carmen Mohan was that she also considered my history of migraines and sleep issues. With that information, she prescribed a single medication that addressed all three concerns—anxiety, migraines, and sleep. It was such a relief to add just one prescription to my daily life instead of three.

It took several weeks to notice a difference, but it was truly life-changing. My biggest symptom before the medication was rumination. Anxiety rumination is the cognitive process of repeatedly dwelling on negative thoughts, experiences, or emotions. For me, it felt like my brain was stuck in a constant doom scroll, and it was exhausting: *Did I make my client mad? Is my husband falling out of love with me? Is Tawnya upset with me?* And then, one day, it just stopped. My brain was quiet. It no longer latched on to every negative experience or interaction. My first thought was, *Is this what my brain is supposed to feel like?* Yes, Meagan, this is what a normal brain "sounds" like—master of the obvious.

In 2024, I added counseling to my self-care plan. As I've shared before, I am in the midst of navigating my parents' aging and slowly losing one of my two best friends. To find the right counselor, I asked several colleagues (thank you, Jenay Hicks) for recommendations and ended up interviewing Angela. We talked for about forty-five minutes, and I knew she was the right fit. I used many of the questions outlined above in that consultation.

During the call, I found out she specialized in issues related to grief and loss as well as the development of a nurturing and supportive relationship with the self. She used a systematic approach, and with my brain, I needed someone to help me name what I was feeling and put a process in place for me to work through my complicated feelings intentionally.

At first, we met weekly so I could learn tools to help me manage my "new normal." I cried through most of those first sessions, unable to regulate my emotions. Now, we meet every three to four weeks, but I know she'll make space for me if I need her sooner.

There are other things that are vital to my mental health, like yoga and running. Yoga has been shown to reduce anxiety and depression by calming the nervous system and lowering stress hormones. A Harvard Health study notes that just as lifting weights strengthens your muscles, practicing yoga strengthens your brain. It promotes the formation of new neural connections and improves cognitive functions such as learning and memory. It also fortifies regions of the brain responsible for attention, awareness, thought, language, and memory. In many ways, yoga is like weight training for your mind.[27]

Most days, you'll find me in row three at Sacred Thread Yoga, often with tears running down my face. Yes, I'm "that" girl—but the community understands that this is how I work through complicated emotions and gives me the space I need. They know what I do for a living and a bit about the people in my life. It's cathartic, and I always leave with a sense of quiet calm, feeling lighter and more connected to my body.

Running is also part of my mental health practice. It serves as a moving meditation, helping me tune in to my body, focus on my breath, and concentrate only on the next step. Admittedly, I HATE the first ten to fifteen minutes of every run, but once I get past that, I feel good and settled. And boy did I miss it this October. We returned from a week in London, and my body rebelled. It took two weeks to recover from a sinus infection and whatever other crud I had. I could not run for almost three weeks, which affected me both mentally and physically.

Thankfully, I am back at it again, albeit for shorter distances for now as I work my way back to my previous shape.

You might be wondering, *Why is she sharing all this?* Because there are so many different tools that can support mental health. I want to empower you to choose the ones that make the most sense for you. Below is my personal list of tools and activities that have helped me boost and protect my own mental health:

SLEEP	**MEDITATION**	**MINDFULNESS**
Journaling	Practicing gratitude	Exercise
Yoga	Counseling	Going outside
Humming (yes, really)	Sitting in the sun	Breathing exercises
Talking to a friend	Calm app (sleep stories)	Peloton app (running, meditation)
Oura Ring	Support groups	

These aren't magic solutions or one-size-fits-all prescriptions—they're simply the practices that have supported me as I navigate the messy, unpredictable landscape of anticipatory grief. Your list might look similar or might be completely different, and that's exactly the point. What matters is not *what* you choose but rather that you choose something that helps you feel steadier, softer, or even just 1 percent more grounded on any given day. Let this be an invitation to keep exploring, keep listening to your body, and keep giving yourself permission to care for your whole self—mind, body, and spirit—as you walk this path.

Part III

COPING, CONNECTING, AND FINDING MEANING

Chapter 6

BEING PRESENT DURING THE FEAR

"Presence doesn't erase fear—it gives fear somewhere to rest."

Anticipatory grief often lives in the tension between *knowing* and *not knowing*. You may know that something difficult is coming, yet you don't know when, how, or what life will look like after it happens. That uncertainty can make it nearly impossible to stay in the present. The mind races ahead: *What will happen next? How much time do we have? Will I be okay when they're gone?*

The truth is that the moments that will sustain you later—the ones you'll return to again and again—are happening right now. Learning to stay in them, even briefly, is an act of courage. Fear is an inevitable part of the grieving process. This chapter will help you remain present when fear surges—by tending to your nervous system, protecting your relationships, and creating small, sustainable rituals that bring meaning over time.

Being present during anticipatory grief isn't about denying fear; it's about holding it gently. When we resist fear, it grows louder. When we acknowledge it, the edges soften. Greg does this by focusing on today: "I do not know what is going to happen in the future, but I do know we have today."

In my work with clients—and in my own experience with Staci—I've learned that presence can be practiced in micro-moments. You don't need an hour of meditation or a weekend retreat to find stillness. You need one breath. One pause. One act of noticing. Sometimes, it's placing a hand on your chest before walking into the hospital room to feel your heartbeat or taking three slow breaths while sitting in the car after a long appointment. It might be noticing the way your loved one's shoulders relax when you hold their hand or letting yourself really taste the first sip of coffee in the morning before the day rushes in. These tiny moments don't change the reality you're living in, but they create just enough space for your nervous system to settle—and for you to remember that you're still here, still breathing, still connected.

Presence begins in the body. When the mind is spinning, the body becomes the anchor. During sessions, I often remind clients that their bodies can help calm their minds. Practitioners of mindfulness frequently say, "Calm body, calm mind." And now, science confirms that this connection is more than a metaphor.

A study from the Washington University School of Medicine in St. Louis found that regions of the brain responsible for movement are linked to networks involved in thinking, planning, and regulating automatic functions like heart rate and blood pressure.[28] In other words, the brain's very structure reveals a tangible connection between body and mind—showing that how we move and how we think are deeply intertwined.

This research also helps explain why anxiety makes some people pace, why stimulating the vagus nerve through deep belly breathing can ease depression, and why regular exercise improves mood and outlook. Science is clear: Tending to the body is one of the most effective ways to support the mind.

Self-Care Practices for Anticipatory Grief

With this understanding, let's begin with self-care—because caring for your body and for your emotional well-being are inseparable.

There are many myths about self-care, so let's level with this definition: **Self-care** is the intentional pursuit of integrated wellness—balancing mind, body, and spirit, both personally and professionally.

Self-care goes far beyond physical health. Running or meditation might be great for some people, but if you dread doing them, they aren't truly self-care for you. The most meaningful practices are those that energize, soothe, or fulfill you—activities you look forward to.

Still, many people feel conflicted about self-care. Culturally, we don't promote it. In the United States, work has become a status symbol, and exhaustion often passes as a badge of honor. *Harvard Business Review* notes that "busy" has become our default response to "How are you?"—a reflection of how deeply we equate busyness with worth.[29]

This mindset colors how we approach rest, time off, and even self-compassion. We sometimes view kindness toward ourselves as indulgent or unproductive. For many people, their inner dialogue sounds like: *I'll rest when everything else is done, I shouldn't need a break—other people have it worse,* or *If I step away, everything will fall apart, and it will be my fault.* Some tell themselves, *I'm being lazy* simply for wanting an afternoon off, or *I don't deserve a vacation until I've earned it* even when they're exhausted. But these beliefs can quietly block our ability to care for ourselves at all. True self-care requires not just intention but permission to believe that your well-being matters as much as your productivity. Because in the long run, it does.

Here are some of the top myths about self-care:

Myth 1: "Self-care is selfish."

- Truth: Tending to your body and mind preserves your capacity to love and advocate.
- Reframe: "Rest is relationship maintenance."
- Try this: Schedule a twenty-minute "care block" after hard appointments (a walk, a nap, or a cup of tea). Put it on the calendar like a medical prescription or appointment.

Myth 2: "If I'm okay, I'm not grieving hard enough."

- Truth: Nervous systems oscillate. Windows of okayness are healthy, not disloyal.
- Reframe: "Stability is fuel for the next wave."
- Try this: Keep a "permission note" in your phone: *It's safe to enjoy this hour.*

Myth 3: "Self-care fixes feelings."

- Truth: It regulates feelings, but it doesn't erase them.
- Reframe: "I'm lowering the volume, not muting the station."
- Try this: Rate your distress from zero to ten before and after an activity. Celebrate a one- to two-point shift.

Myth 4: "I don't have time."

- Truth: Micro-practices (30–120 seconds) change physiology.
- Reframe: "Small and done daily beats big and done rarely."
- Try this: Pair a sixty-second grounding exercise like box breathing with an existing routine (handwashing, unlocking the door).

Myth 5: "Boundaries make me cold."

- Truth: Boundaries protect connection from overload.
- Reframe: "Boundaries are how love lasts."
- Try this: "I can talk for fifteen minutes now or tomorrow afternoon for longer—what's better for you?"

Please take a minute to write down your own misgivings about self-care. Once that is completed, how can you reframe them?

Mindfulness Practices for Anticipatory Grief

Mindfulness is a powerful way to build emotional and cognitive skills that help you navigate anticipatory grief. In my view, it is also a profound form of self-care.

So what is **mindfulness**? At its core, mindfulness is the practice of paying attention to the present moment with gentle, nonjudgmental awareness. It invites you to notice your thoughts, feelings, bodily sensations, and surroundings without becoming swept away by them. Mindfulness can look like feeling your feet on the ground while waiting in line at the pharmacy, noticing the warmth of your coffee mug before the day ramps up, or observing the rise and fall of your breath when you feel anxiety tightening your chest. It might be pausing long enough to recognize, *Wow, I'm really overwhelmed right now* and, instead of pushing past it, taking ten seconds to name the sounds you hear in the room when your mind starts racing.

Mindfulness can also be incredibly simple:

- Placing a hand over your belly when a difficult emotion surfaces, noticing the subtle rise and fall beneath your palm.
- Taking one conscious inhale before answering a hard question or making a medical decision.
- Noticing the sensation of water on your skin during a shower instead of mentally rehearsing the worst-case scenario.
- Eating the first bite of a meal slowly, feeling the texture and taste before the autopilot of worry returns.
- Letting your shoulders drop when you realize they've been sitting next to your ears for hours.

- Naming what is true in the moment—"My chest feels tight," "My jaw is clenched," "I'm scared"—without trying to fix it right away.
- Looking out a window for twenty seconds, paying attention to the movement of trees or passing clouds, to remind your body that the world outside your fear is still turning.

These small practices help you create space between stimulus and response—so that instead of reacting automatically, you can respond with intention and calm. Amid a grief journey when so much feels uncontrollable, mindfulness becomes a way of reclaiming even a sliver of agency, grounding you in the one place your body always knows how to return to: this moment, right here, right now.

Research continues to show that mindfulness isn't just a spiritual or emotional exercise—it has measurable effects on the brain and body. A growing body of evidence from neuroscience demonstrates that regular mindfulness practice can reduce activity in the amygdala (the brain's fear center) while strengthening the prefrontal cortex, which is responsible for emotional regulation and executive function.[30]

A landmark study from Harvard University found that just eight weeks of mindfulness training led to measurable increases in gray matter density in areas of the brain associated with learning, memory, empathy, and stress regulation.[31] Another meta-analysis published in *JAMA Internal Medicine* reviewed more than forty clinical trials and concluded that mindfulness-based interventions significantly reduced anxiety, depression, and perceived stress.[32]

Physiologically, mindfulness supports the body's ability to recover from chronic stress. Studies have shown that it lowers cortisol levels, improves immune function, and even supports cardiovascular health by helping regulate blood pressure and heart rate variability.

For individuals living with anticipatory grief, these benefits are especially meaningful. Mindfulness can help you tolerate uncertainty, manage intrusive thoughts, and reconnect with small, grounding moments of peace. It doesn't erase the pain—but it teaches you how to sit with it without being consumed by it. In real life, this might look like noticing your breath instead of spiraling into panic while waiting for a scan result or placing a hand on your heart when your mind leaps to worst-case scenarios. It can be sitting at your loved one's bedside and intentionally feeling the warmth of their hand instead of bracing for the moment it might be gone. It might mean acknowledging, *Right now we're okay* during an unexpectedly calm afternoon or grounding yourself by feeling your feet on the floor when grief threatens to pull you into the future. These practices don't change what's coming, but they help you stay anchored to the moments you still have.

I have outlined several mindfulness practices that can easily be integrated into your daily life. Each is brief and, when practiced consistently, can reduce stress, increase self-compassion, and strengthen your capacity to be present with the many emotions of anticipatory grief.

The Sixty-Second Drop

This is a one-minute nervous system reset. It uses quick body and breath cues to shift you from fight or flight toward a steadier focus. This exercise will help you feel grounded, and by releasing common tension spots in your jaw and shoulders, it mitigates the body's threat alarm.

- Feel your feet.
- Soften the jaw/shoulders.
- Inhale for the count of four, exhale for the count of six (five rounds like this).
- Name it: "I'm safe at this moment."
- Use: Before entering a room, answering a call, or starting paperwork.

5-4-3-2-1 Senses Reset

The 5-4-3-2-1 technique is one of the easiest mindfulness strategies, designed for managing stress and anxiety. This simple exercise can be done almost anywhere and at any time. It's also one of the most effective since it uses the five senses to ground you in the present moment.

- Name five things you can see, four you can feel, three you can hear, two you can smell, and one you can taste.
- Use: In waiting rooms, in parking lots, during midnight spirals.

The Worry Window

The Worry Window is one of my favorite cognitive behavioral techniques. It is one of the most frequent go-to exercises that I use with my clients. To use the technique, you simply need to set aside an allotted amount of time to worry. At this time, it is essential to get everything you are worried about out of your head and onto a piece of paper. It also helps set you boundaries with your worries, since you know you have an appointment with yourself when they will get 100 percent of your attention.

- Set a daily fifteen-minute window to list worries. If you find yourself worrying outside of that window, jot them down and say, "I'll meet you at 7 p.m."
- Use: To keep fear acknowledged but bounded, during middle-of-the-night ruminations.

A worry window gives my anxious brain its own tiny office with a door I can close. It's just me, my notebook, and whatever fear decided to tap me on the shoulder that day. Getting the thoughts out of my head and onto paper creates a boundary—a way of saying, "You get your fifteen minutes, but you do *not* get the whole day." And honestly, knowing I have an appointment with myself later makes it easier to stay present with the actual humans in my life. Because when I'm not mentally wrestling with my runaway thoughts, I have more space to connect—to laugh with a friend, actually listen to Tim, or be fully with Staci instead of spiraling three steps ahead in my imagination.

As you build your own self-care practices that help you navigate anticipatory grief—whether that's a daily worry window, journaling, or simply getting your thoughts out of your head and onto paper (or into a notes app on your phone)—you also create more space for connection in real life. When your mind feels less cluttered and your nervous system is less overwhelmed, you're better able to show up with presence for the people who matter.

Self-care isn't selfish or separate from connection; it's what allows you to engage more deeply. Once you've tended to your internal landscape, you can begin creating intentional moments of connection that will support you throughout this season.

Creating Intentional Moments of Connection

When someone you love is ill—or when life feels fragile—big gestures often give way to small ones. Grand plans dissolve into tiny, sacred moments: a shared cup of tea, a photo of sunlight on a windowsill, a text that simply says "Thinking of you."

Staci and I started calling these our "micro-moments." They're small enough to fit into even the most challenging days. Sometimes, they're as simple as swapping favorite songs from Taylor Swift's new album or good morning texts. Micro-moments don't erase fear, but they make it bearable. They tether us to something real—proof that life continues to offer beauty, even in the hard times.

Try planning one micro-moment each day:

- Sharing meaningful quotes via Instagram (Staci and I do this on a daily basis).
- Taking a photograph of something that represents resilience.
- Spending a few minutes in shared silence, hand in hand.
- Listening to a playlist of songs that mean something to you both (we included one at the end for you).

What matters is not the act itself but the *attention* you bring to it.

Small Rituals, Big Meaning

Rituals give shape to chaos. They remind us that even as things change, we can still choose intention. Some rituals may emerge naturally; others you may need to create deliberately. Over time, they become part of the fabric of your relationship—anchors that mark your care and presence. By making small acts of meaning—lighting a candle, writing a letter, sharing a memory with someone—we carve out a safe space where our grief, our fear, our longing can be seen and felt rather than ignored.

Almost every day, I complete a ritual that reminds me of Staci. She made me a friendship bracelet that says "bestie." When I put it on, it makes me smile and makes me automatically think about her. It brings comfort on hard days when time feels too fleeting. It's part of a stack of bracelets I wear routinely: "breathe" from my mom, and "badass" and "be brave" from me to me.

Rituals also help us slow down and honor what was and what still is. On a practical level, they restore a sense of control, provide structure in a moment of hardship, and help us connect to others or to something bigger than ourselves. Here are some you might consider:

- **Shared playlist:** Create a playlist for treatment days. Include songs that make you both laugh, cry, or breathe deeper. We made a chemo playlist for Staci; you can find it on Spotify and in the Appendix.
- **A gratitude jar:** Each week, write down one small thing you're grateful for and drop it in a jar. Read them together when energy allows.
- **Tree or garden ritual:** Plant something living—something that will continue to grow.
- **Meaningful tokens:** Exchange small objects that remind you of one another—a friendship bracelet, a photograph, a quote. These can travel between you when words feel heavy.

Rituals aren't just symbolic—they're healing. Studies show they can reduce anxiety, restore a sense of control, and help people process loss more effectively.[33, 34] Rituals remind us that even in the hardest seasons, we still have agency—and the power to create meaning.

When the Fear Feels Too Loud

Presence doesn't mean peace all the time. There are days when fear will still roar and rattle your foundation. When that happens, know that you haven't failed. The goal isn't to *stay* in the present perfectly—it's to return, again and again, with compassion.

If your body feels flooded—racing heart, shallow breath—pause. Name what's happening:

"Fear is here. My mind is scared.
My body is trying to protect me."

And then take one grounding breath. Sometimes, that's enough.

But on the days when fear digs in its heels and refuses to budge, it helps to have a simple, repeatable plan—a way to gently guide yourself back to center when your nervous system wants to sprint into the future. That's where this next tool comes in.

Putting It Together: A Fear-Surge Protocol (Two to Five Minutes)

1. **Stop:** Stop. Take one slow breath. Observe one body sensation. Proceed on purpose.
2. **Ground:** 5-4-3-2-1 or box breathing.
3. **Name and normalize:** "My brain is protecting me; this is anticipatory grief."

4. **Choose one value-action:** Text a check-in, step outside for sixty seconds, fill a water bottle, or start the tea kettle.
5. **Connect:** If you're with your person, say, "Fear's visiting; I'm staying."

STACI

I have the biggest, baddest, most beautiful village. They've shown up for Greg and me in ways I couldn't have imagined. They have delivered meaning right to our door. Meagan jumped in immediately and built a text chain for my posse, started a CaringBridge site, and set up a meal train. She just knew those would help, and she was right. Having one place for updates meant I didn't have to retell hard news a dozen times; it spared my energy for the living I still needed to do. And the meals? They nourished us far beyond calories. When nothing tastes good and decision fatigue is real, not having to think about dinner makes the world a million times easier. And I have been able to use these tools as a platform for asking for help. I was begrudgingly cooking dinner the night after chemo last week and thought, WOW, I could ask for help on the meal train, and people responded immediately.

Love has come in all forms. Cards and gifts are stacked in our house like proof that we are seen. I call it "cancer Christmas." My sister-in-law curated a chemo bag and a prayer blanket from a friend who beat cancer and wrapped me in other people's hope. My dear friend got me a signed copy of Judy Blume's Are You There God? It's Me, Margaret *as recognition of my work. Board chairs who became like family delivered witches' sage and even a tiny voodoo doll from New Orleans, humor and ritual sharing the same shelf. Another package had new underwear, and we laughed until the fear loosened its grip. Cards came from people I don't know; prayers arrived from all faiths. It's impossible to measure the impact of being remembered by strangers, how it lifts the room and your spirit. I even got a box to keep all my cards in, which sits out in the open so I am reminded to revisit those expressions of love often.*

Being present during the fear has also meant honoring my limits, including the boundaries that make care safer. My room is my refuge; my port access is my consent. The people who knock, ask, wait, and accept "not now" are the ones who help me feel at home in my own body. Presence isn't just showing up; it's showing up with respect.

I'm learning to find meaning in movement and in stillness. Sometimes, that looks like getting out of town for a day, hiking at a very slow pace under trees, or standing beside water until it drowns out the ringing in my ears. Sometimes, it's a slow morning in my cave, the sanctuary built by friends, with sun shining in, blankets, music, and permission to do nothing. I tell the story of that space to myself often: You deserve a room where your fear can sit without taking over.

When I can, I do the things I love. Cooking is one of them, even though, right now, everything tastes like GARBAGE. The flavors may be muted, but the ritual still matters—chopping, stirring, feeding the people I love. It's an act of defiance against numbness, a way to stay in the scene of my own life.

Presence, for me, is not a perfect calm; it's a practice of returning. I return to quiet when the noise spikes. I return to my people when loneliness grows loud. I return to the small anchors—the text threads, the smell of a candle, my favorite song—that remind me I'm still here. There is meaning in every moment; my job is to do the work of looking for it. Some days, that's easier than it sounds. Other days, it's a muscle I must consciously flex. Either way, I keep practicing because being present during the fear is how I keep living inside this life I love.

* * *

Our friendship deepened in ways neither of us could have anticipated. Before her diagnosis, Staci and I had the kind of friendship built on shared values, caring deeply about justice, funny texts, hard conversations, and the quiet trust that grows over the years. We could talk about anything—from leadership and purpose to the best way to spend a Saturday morning. But once illness entered the picture, our conversations shifted. They became slower, more intentional, and somehow more alive.

Staci has also gotten better at asking for what she needs.

As I write this, it is November 2025. Today, I got a text that asked me for time this week and if I could take her to chemo on November 6. She has made plans for us for the rest of the year, and Tim and I want to honor her and commit to them. How much time will we have? I don't want any regrets, so we will live big and loud for the rest of 2025, making gingerbread cookies, celebrating her birthday at Argosy Pub with her village, and heading to Highlands, North Carolina, for a few days after Christmas. These moments give us something to look toward, something to anchor ourselves to when so much feels uncertain.

And yet, even with plans on the calendar, each day brings its own mix of challenges and small triumphs. Life doesn't pause for grief; it simply folds around it. To show you what I mean, here's a glimpse into a single week from my journal—a week that captures the emotional whiplash of caring, hoping, coping, and continuing.

November 5, 2025

I went to Pilates. I am out of the house for only an hour. My dad texts that the hematologist wants to do a bone marrow biopsy. That can't be good, and I immediately go into a tailspin. Everything is scheduled around taking care of Becky so much that I worry he isn't taking care of himself. At what point do I say something?

November 6, 2025

Went with Staci to chemo. We talked about the book, Amy, and how she is feeling. I tried to keep things light, even with all the worries about my dad spinning in the back of my mind. Her prognosis looks surprisingly positive—maybe even a few years. But we'll be living scan to scan, six weeks at a time, which only adds to the roller coaster feel of everything.

November 12, 2025

Good day today. Why? I got to lead a wellness workshop for ten human resources leaders with the NFL. The NFL!!! It was the first time the content was entirely mine, not cowritten with anyone else. The presentation focused on small micro-changes leaders can make to take care of themselves and make work and home more sustainable. The women were serious bosses! I was most proud of the fact that, walking into the presentation, I didn't listen to my anxiety. I quietly said to myself, "You are going to crush this," and I did.

November 15, 2025

Staci and Greg came over to watch the Georgia Bulldogs kick Texas's ass in football. Delightful and fun evening, screaming "Go Dawgs" so loud the entire neighborhood could hear. I mean, you didn't want your kids asleep at 11 p.m., did you?

November 17, 2025

Today was a hard day emotionally. At the end of the day, Staci sent me a link to a new movie called *Come See Me in the Good Light*, which came out on Apple TV three days ago. It follows a poet and her partner after she receives a terminal diagnosis. Staci wants to watch it together. I could not even make it through the short trailer without sobbing—literally so hard my body was convulsing. How do I get through these days?

* * *

As a counselor, I was used to helping others name their pain, sit with discomfort, and find meaning in uncertainty. But with Staci, those professional instincts met something far more personal. I am not her therapist. I am her friend, one who carries both clinical knowledge and a broken heart. I found myself learning in real time what I had spent years teaching my clients: that anticipatory grief is not a concept but an experience. It's the quiet rebellion of choosing to love someone fully, knowing that love will one day break your heart.

We've learned to create meaning without forcing it. Sometimes, meaning looks like swapping books. Sometimes, it looks like naming what we're both afraid of out loud and realizing we're still okay in the same room with that truth. Yesterday, it was Staci sharing a trailer for a show on Apple TV called *Come See Me in the Good Light*, referenced above, which chronicles the terminal diagnosis of a poet laureate with ovarian cancer. I cried, and Staci did the same in her world. She bravely asked if I would watch the whole movie with her, and of course, I said yes. I know that when we do, it will break something open in both of us—but we will find our footing together. Maybe it will be a dress rehearsal for what's coming. Perhaps it will be preparation. Or maybe it will simply be an acknowledgment of what's to come.

I once asked Staci how she stays grounded through treatment and the hard that comes with it. She said, "I try to make meaning in the moment, not in the outcome." That sentence stays with me. Walking with Staci through her illness changed how I understand both grief and healing. It stripped away the distance between theory and reality, between counselor and friend. It reminded me that love is, at its core, an act of courage. And that sometimes, the most profound thing we can do for someone is simply to stay—to keep showing up, even when there are no answers left to give.

Journaling Exercises

- Where did fear show up in my body today? What softened it, even 10 percent?

- What micro-ritual felt nourishing? What will I repeat this week?

- Design one small ritual you can begin today.

- What feels meaningful or grounding for you right now?

- How can you bring a moment of connection or gratitude into your daily routine?

- Who can you invite into that moment with you?

What Success Looks Like (Realistically)

Success in grief and presence isn't about eliminating hard emotions—it's about finding your way back to steadiness more quickly each time you're knocked off-balance. It's not about perfect conversations or always knowing the right thing to say but about creating more intentional moments of connection, even in the midst of fear. And it's not measured in grand gestures or dramatic breakthroughs but in the small, repeatable rituals that fit inside real life—the daily acts of showing up, breathing together, and remembering that love still lives here. These are the threads that hold us when everything else feels uncertain. And in the chapters that follow, you'll see how these quiet practices come to life through the stories of other people—ordinary moments that reveal extraordinary truths about what it means to love someone through a season of anticipatory grief.

Chapter 7

THE POWER OF STORY

"Grief doesn't end the story. It changes who tells it."

Storytelling is one of the oldest forms of healing. Across cultures and centuries, people have gathered around fires, in churches, on porches, and now in digital spaces to make sense of loss through words. When someone we love is facing illness or decline, storytelling becomes both a matter of survival and a legacy—a way to hold on to meaning when everything else feels uncertain.

For those living through anticipatory grief, stories tether us to life. They allow us to transform fear into connection and helplessness into contribution. Telling the story—theirs, yours, and the shared one between you—helps shape what remains. It's what Staci and I are doing right now with this book.

Why Telling the Story Matters

There are three reasons storytelling becomes so powerful during anticipatory grief: for them, for you, and for legacy. For your loved one, storytelling helps preserve identity when illness or decline begins to take pieces of them away. Sharing memories, milestones, and even everyday moments reminds them—and you—of who they are beyond the diagnosis. For you, storytelling provides a way to process what's happening in real time. Talking about memories or writing them down gives shape to emotions that might otherwise feel too heavy or chaotic to carry. And for legacy, storytelling becomes a bridge between past, present, and future. These stories outlive the moment, becoming threads that keep the connection alive after the loss. In this way, storytelling transforms grief from something that feels isolating into something that honors, connects, and continues.

For Them

When someone is navigating a serious illness or nearing the end of life, being witnessed and seen matters; your loved one's story deserves to be told in their own words, on their own terms. Many people fear being remembered only for their illness—the diagnosis that overshadows the decades of life that came before it. Inviting them to tell their story is an act of restoration. It says, "You are more than what's happening to your body or mind."

Ask them about their childhood—the tree they used to climb, the teacher who believed in them, the trouble they got into with their siblings. Ask about the music that shaped their early years, the song they danced to at their wedding, or the tune they still hum without thinking. Invite them to share the proudest moments of their life: the first job that made them feel capable, the day they became a parent, the moment they realized they were truly loved. Record the sound of their laughter or the way they tell a familiar story. Sit with them as they choose which photos to place by their bedside or which family recipes they hope will outlive them. Let them decide what memories to keep alive. Help them make meaning, not by forcing reflection but by holding space for the pieces of their life that still feel whole, beautiful, and deeply theirs.

For You

Telling your version of the story—the caregiving, the waiting, the sacred moments—is just as important. It helps you process emotions, transforming what's overwhelming into something you can hold and eventually cherish. Maybe it's naming the exhaustion of setting an alarm every three hours to give medication or describing the way you memorized the pattern of your loved one's breathing during long hospital nights. Maybe it's remembering the tenderness of brushing their hair, the quiet humor in choosing the "good" blanket for chemo days, or the relief of hearing them say, "I'm glad you're here." These details matter.

When we give language to experience, we reclaim a sense of agency. Writing or speaking about the story doesn't erase the pain, but it organizes the memories—like placing scattered puzzle pieces into an image you can finally make sense of. Your story reminds you that you've been brave, that you've loved deeply, and that even in grief, you are still growing. You are all reading Staci's and my storytelling in these pages, witnessing how the messy, tender details become a record not just of loss but of connection, courage, and care.

For Legacy

Legacy isn't about perfection or performance; it's about preservation. Stories become bridges for those who will come after your loved one is gone—family, friends, or communities who may one day face similar loss. Through story, we pass on lessons about what it means to love, to care, to let go, and to live fully even when life feels fragile. When we tell stories aloud, we turn grief into something communal. It is also an excellent way for future generations to know the person who has passed away. Imagine your newborn hearing her grandfather's recorded voice. Or your son using his great-grandmother's chili recipe. One of my most treasured rituals is making my great-aunt Margaret's homemade chicken soup. It has become a staple in the cold winter months—not just because it's soup but because it brings back the memories we shared. She let me stay up way past bedtime to watch *The Love Boat* and *Fantasy Island*. Her house had the coolest organ, filled with buttons that added bass, snare, or even a calypso beat. Aunt Margaret let me touch everything and allowed my imagination to run wild. It's funny how something as simple as making soup can bring back treasured memories.

These small points of connection keep the legacy alive. By telling these stories and sharing rituals and family traditions, we also allow others to tell theirs too. Grief does not need to be hidden or silenced.

Stories from Others Living in the In-Between

Throughout my work, I've heard countless stories from people navigating anticipatory grief. As we move deeper into meaning-making, it's important to remember that healing doesn't always mean returning to who we were before. Sometimes, it means becoming someone new in the aftermath of what we've endured.

Dr. William Walker

Dr. William Walker's story captures that kind of courage. He was a twenty-seven-year-old medical student used to exhaustion, skipped meals, and one-hundred-hour workweeks. Fatigue and weight loss felt like part of the training. But when a cough made him feel like he was drowning and a lump appeared on his neck, he knew something was wrong. Within weeks, he heard the words that would split his life into before and after:

"You have cancer."

His first reaction wasn't fear—it was relief. Finally, an answer. In the late 1980s, when AIDS was a death sentence, cancer felt like a "fighting chance." He joked later that his biggest surprise wasn't the diagnosis but how much medicine he didn't know. "Everything was paper charts, missed orders, and waiting. Maybe one day AI will cure it," he laughed.

Humor became his lifeline. When doctors injected dye between his toes for staging, they promised it would feel like a "pinprick." He said, "That hurt more than anything you can imagine." Then he looked down at his green-stained feet and his crooked belly button scar and smiled. "The trivia we obsess over."

That kind of laughter wasn't denial; it was resistance—a way to stay human in the face of the unthinkable. But beneath the humor ran a deep spiritual surrender. When his fever spiked to 107 degrees and doctors wanted to intubate him, he refused. "If my higher power wants me to keep walking this earth, I will."

Later, during that delirious night, he saw a bright light and heard, "You have to go back. It's not time yet." He did go back to medicine, to life, to purpose. Yet the story didn't end with remission. Decades later, at fifty-two, the long-term side effects of chemotherapy left him permanently disabled. The treatment that saved his life ultimately altered it again, forcing him to grieve a second time—not for death but for his life before endless fatigue, the loss of cognition, and the end of a career he once enjoyed.

Let me explain: A 1990s St. Jude study on acute lymphoblastic leukemia (ALL) treated with a chemotherapy-only protocol found that patients had a statistically significant higher risk of below-average performance in sustained attention, processing speed, and academic abilities.[35] This protocol showed that chemotherapy can impact cognitive function. A study published in the *Journal of the National Cancer Institute* in 2022 confirmed these findings.[36] This is what Dr. Walker experienced in the years following his treatment, leading to his long-term disability.

For Dr. Walker, grief carried anger, frustration, disbelief, humor, and faith all at once. It was never a single emotion but a mosaic of them—the human attempt to make meaning when life changes course. His story reminds us that healing doesn't mean life returns to what it was; it means learning to live fully in what remains.

Tools for Recording Memories

There's no right way to capture a story. The only rule is this: Do it in a way that feels natural and true to the person you love. Here are a few examples that help families and loved ones preserve meaning and connection.

Audio Journals

Record short conversations or spontaneous reflections using your phone or a voice memo app. Capture the sound of laughter, favorite sayings, or simple details like what song is playing in the background. Ask your dad to record a lullaby for your future children to listen to or save a simple "I love you" that you can pull up anytime. A voice holds a texture that words on a page can't replicate.

I've started stockpiling voicemails myself—my mom calling just to say, "I love you," or my dad leaving a message saying he's "so grateful for Tim's and my help." These tiny audio snapshots become anchors, things to return to when you need their presence in a way only a voice can provide.

Letters and Legacy Notes

Write letters to or with your loved one. They can be short—"One thing I've always wanted to tell you is . . ." or "My favorite memory with you is . . ." Encourage them to write letters too. These notes later become touchstones, a way to feel their presence on days when silence feels heavy. Staci will share how she is going to have letters delivered to specific people for special events after she has died.

Video Conversations

Film small moments, not just milestones. A cup of coffee, a shared walk, or the retelling of a familiar family story. Consider using gentle prompts:

- What brings you peace?
- What do you hope people remember about you?
- What has love taught you?

Storybooks or Digital Collages

Platforms like StoryCorps and MemoryWell, as well as simple printed photo books, allow you to combine images, quotes, and reflections. The process itself—curating and revisiting—can be healing. My husband, Tim, has done an outstanding job of preserving our memories via Shutterfly books. We get them out at least once a year to share memories of special times we have shared as a couple and with other people we love. I asked him last night to start capturing all our time with Greg and Staci so we can make a book for them and for us.

These practices don't have to be perfect or polished. The purpose isn't production; it's about capturing the authenticity of your connection.

STACI

I've been thinking a lot about what I want to leave behind, and I want to make space for my people to ask for what would be meaningful to them. I tried to do that early on, but I think it was too soon; now, I think we all feel more ready.

To start, I definitely want to write letters for important moments I might miss. I imagine letters to my godson, Ellis, for his graduation, when he finds love, and as he discovers his career path; a letter to Amy, for her wedding or when she buys a home; a letter to Meagan for when Cooper or her mom passes; a letter to my partner, Greg, for when he finds love again.

Beyond letters, someone recently told me I could record my voice and create an AI avatar so that Greg and other loved ones could "talk" with me after I'm gone. I think that's a beautiful idea and a thoughtful way to use technology.

In the same spirit of legacy, Greg bought me a reMarkable tablet early on to make work easier, and I began using it to write a book about my lifelong fight for bodily autonomy and the lessons I've learned along the way. Then Meagan approached me about this project, and I immediately said yes—yes to a cool collaboration with her and yes to anything that might help others walking this path.

On a practical note, I want to inventory the things in our home so Greg knows where they came from and why they matter. Let's be honest: I did the decorating, and he can be less than observant, so a guide would help.

I'm also thinking about keepsakes, my jewelry, and other uniquely "me" items and how to pass them along to the people who would cherish them most. I want to experience the joy of passing those along.

Most importantly, I want to say, "I've had the most amazing life." I hope I remember to say that with my last breath.

Reflection Page: Storytelling as Healing

"When we tell our stories, we make meaning.
When we listen to others, we make connections.
And when we preserve those stories, we make a legacy."

Storytelling is not just about remembering—it's about reconnecting. This reflection page invites you to explore your story, your loved one's story, and the spaces where they intertwine. During anticipatory grief, stories help bridge the distance between what was, what is, and what's coming. They become a way to hold on to love.

This reflection exercise is for you, the reader, to help guide your process as you preserve your loved one's legacy.

Part I: Your Loved One's Story

1. What moments or memories feel most alive when you think about your loved one?
   Try writing sensory details—what you saw, heard, or felt in those moments.

2. How would you describe their essence in a few words?
   Think beyond roles—who are they at their core?

3. What story do they love to tell about themselves or their life?
   Write it down in their words if you can.

4. What story do you want to make sure others remember about them?

Part II: Your Story in This Season

1. How would you describe your own story right now?
   Are you in a chapter of waiting, caregiving, transformation?

2. What parts of your experience have felt too hard—or too sacred—to put into words?
   You don't need to share them; just name them here.

3. What meaning or growth has emerged, even in small ways, through this experience?

Part III: Shared Stories and Legacy

1. What are three small ways you can capture or preserve your shared story?
   ☐ Record a short conversation
   ☐ Write a memory letter
   ☐ Create a photo or video collection
   ☐ Share a story at family gatherings
   ☐ Other: ______________

2. How do humor, joy, or play show up in your relationship —even now?
   Describe a time when you laughed together recently. What did that moment teach you about resilience?

3. What do you hope others will learn from witnessing your story?

Part IV: The Power of Retelling

"Telling the story once helps you survive it. Telling it again helps you understand it."

1. How does it feel to tell your story out loud or on paper? *Notice: Do you feel lighter, sadder, or more connected?*

2. What's one story you're ready to share—with a friend, a therapist, or your journal?

Closing Intention

Write a short intention statement you want to carry forward from this chapter:

"As I move through grief, I will honor the stories that shaped us by _____________."

CHAPTER 8

COMMUNITY, FAITH, AND SUPPORT

Grief is, at its core, an experience of separation—from a person, a relationship, or a future that will no longer exist. That separation doesn't only exist between you and your loved one; it can also create distance between you and the rest of the world. When grief enters a room, it often brings silence and isolation with it.

When someone you love is facing a serious illness, life can begin to shrink. You may notice that people stop calling or don't know what to say. Friends who once felt close may pull away, unsure how to show up. Others may offer well-meaning words that don't land—"You're so strong" or "At least you still have time"—phrases that only widen the gap between what you feel and what they understand. Even surrounded by people, you can feel profoundly alone.

The truth is that no one experiences grief in exactly the same way. Even if others have lived through similar losses, your relationship, your memories, and your pain are uniquely yours. That individuality can make grief feel isolating—as if no one could possibly understand what you're carrying. And in a sense, that's true. Grief is as personal as a fingerprint. But being unique in your experience doesn't mean you must be alone in it.

This kind of isolation can happen to both the caregiver and the person who is ill. Friends may not know what to say or how to show up for you. Invitations become fewer; conversations are shorter. The world retreats right when you need it the most.

Sometimes, isolation is self-protective. When emotions are raw, it can feel safer to pull back—to conserve energy and protect yourself from further misunderstanding or pain. But over time, this quiet withdrawal can deepen the feelings of disconnection.

Isolation amplifies grief. We are wired for coregulation—to steady ourselves by hearing another person's voice, feeling a hand on our shoulder, or simply knowing someone is nearby. Without those cues, the body works harder to manage fear, sadness, and uncertainty on its own.

When we're disconnected from others, our nervous system loses one of its greatest regulators: social connection. Research shows that social isolation and loneliness activate the same neural pathways as physical pain.[37] In fact, brain regions like the dorsal anterior cingulate cortex and anterior insula—the same areas that activate when we stub a toe or break a bone—also light up when we feel excluded, rejected, or alone.[38,39] Imagine that your brain understands that the pain caused by loss is the same as the pain caused by a broken bone. And just a reminder, broken bones don't heal overnight. The body doesn't distinguish between emotional isolation and physical injury; it registers both as threats.

This is why grief feels heavier when you're facing it in silence.

- A simple decision about medication can feel overwhelming without someone to talk it through with.

- The fear of an upcoming scan expands when you're carrying it alone at 2 a.m.
- Even moments of hope can feel disorienting when there's no one to share them with.

Example: Isolation

It's 10:47 p.m. The house is quiet, and the only light is the glow from the kitchen stove clock. You're standing at the sink, gripping the counter, replaying the oncologist's words from earlier that day: *"The scan shows progression."*

You want to talk to someone, but everyone in your life feels far away. You don't want to "burden" your friends, and your family means well, but they always reach for silver linings or the upside you're too tired to hold. So you keep it to yourself. The fear curls tight in your chest. Your thoughts ping-pong between what's coming and what you're not ready to face. Loneliness makes everything louder—the grief, the questions, the what-ifs.

Even the refrigerator humming feels like it's mocking how silent your life has become.

Example: Connection

Now, imagine the same evening, the same news, the same grief—but one thing is different. You text a friend: "Rough scan today. I don't have many words."

Two minutes later, your phone buzzes. "I'm up. You don't have to talk. I'm just here."

You put the phone to your ear and breathe. Neither of you says much. Your friend's steady presence on the other end of the line slows your heartbeat, loosens your shoulders, and makes the room feel less suffocating. You don't talk about hope or outcomes. You just exist in the moment together. The grief is still there—but it's held, not carried alone. The night feels a little more bearable.

In the end, connection doesn't erase the grief or change the reality of what you're facing—but it does change how you carry it. Isolation magnifies fear; connection distributes the weight. Sometimes, that connection comes through deep conversations, and sometimes, it comes through nothing more than a friend's quiet presence on the other end of a phone. Grief will always be heavy, but it becomes more bearable when held in community. Reaching toward others, even in small ways, is not a sign of weakness; it is an act of courage, a reminder that we were never meant to shoulder this alone.

The Healing Power of Humor

Humor may feel out of place in the midst of grief, but it's often the very thing that keeps us going. Grief doesn't erase laughter—it changes its tone. The jokes get darker, the punchlines softer, and the timing sacred. In hospital rooms and waiting areas, I've heard some of the most honest, gut-level laughter of my life. It's not denial; it's survival. Researchers have found that humor can actually buffer stress by releasing endorphins and lowering cortisol levels.[40] In other words, a well-timed laugh doesn't just lighten the mood—it recalibrates the body. It signals safety to the nervous system . . . and God knows we can all use that.

Many caregivers describe "gallows humor" as their secret coping strategy: finding absurdity in IV pumps that beep like a Michael Jackson tune or laughing when someone accidentally brings kale chips to a chemo appointment instead of comfort snacks. It's not making light of pain—it's making space for breath.

In my own work and in conversations with people like Staci, I've learned that humor often takes the edge off the challenging moments. It reminds us that we are still alive, still capable of feeling something beyond grief. The last time I went to chemo with Staci, we were talking to one of the nurses about one of the drugs Staci was getting.

Actually, I'm going to tell this story myself. One of the drugs I get with chemo is a steroid called Decadron. The first time I got it was the day I got my port, and I had SO MANY drugs during the course of surgery, then chemo in the same day. When the nurse was administering the Decadron, I asked, "Is it normal for my labia and butt to be itchy?" She responded, "Oh, I need to slow down. We call that 'ants in the pants.' It comes on if the drug is pushed too fast." Let me tell you, those are some specific ants in some very specific parts of your pants. When I later got that drug again at chemo with Meagan, we were telling the infusion nurse that story. That nurse then told us about the first time she'd administered Decadron and no one had told her to go slow. So imagine what a male patient would do if his penis suddenly felt as if it were on fire! We all cackled so hard.

Sometimes, the kindest thing we can do for ourselves—or for someone we love—is to let a small laugh cut through the heaviness. Laughter is just one way we can connect with others.

Connection is not a luxury in grief; it's a lifeline. Just as the body needs rest, hydration, and nourishment, the grieving heart needs contact, understanding, and witness. Without it, pain has nowhere to go—it circulates inward, tightening until it turns into numbness or despair.

As I've shared before, I often retreat into solitude when I'm sad and have learned that it isn't helpful for me emotionally or mentally. Earlier this year, after one of my dad's more difficult medical updates, I came home, put my phone on silent, and crawled into bed fully clothed. I told myself I was "fine," but really, I was shutting down. I didn't answer when friends reached out; I didn't tell Tim what was wrong. I just folded in on myself, hoping the quiet would soften the blow. Instead, the silence made the fear louder. So I pushed through the pain and called Tawnya.

Tawnya is my other best friend, someone who has known me since I was twenty-four. How is that possible? She is also a badass. She has a serious big girl job—the chief commercial officer of ViaPlus by VINCI Highways. By the time I got off the phone with her, I was in tears from laughing so hard. Those few minutes of real, honest connection helped pull me out of my shell and push me back into the world with a bit more energy and much steadier footing. When pain is witnessed, it becomes shared, and when it's shared, it becomes lighter. I promise.

Finding Community in the Midst of Loss

When someone you love is facing a serious illness, life can begin to shrink. Hospital schedules, treatment routines, and emotional exhaustion rearrange your world. The social life that once kept you balanced—wine club, pickleball, book club, or a simple girls' night—fades into the background. You may notice that people stop calling or don't know what to say.

Support groups are often one of the most powerful spaces for this kind of shared experience. In a room of strangers who "get it," you may find yourself breathing a little easier. There's relief in not having to explain why specific dates are harder or why laughter and tears can coexist. In a support group, you might hear someone say, "I also sit in my car for twenty minutes before going into the hospital," and feel your shoulders drop because you suddenly realize you're not the only one. Someone else might share the guilt of feeling relief after a loved one passes, and instead of judgment, the group nods in recognition. Another person may offer a practical tip—like keeping a "go bag" in the car for long clinic days—or talk openly about the loneliness of being the only sibling doing the caregiving.

In online groups, support can look like a middle-of-the-night post that simply says, "I can't sleep; I'm scared," and within minutes, someone replies, "You're not alone. I'm here too." It might be people swapping stories about the small things keeping them going—favorite snacks, playlists for long drives, or the ritual of getting Dunkin Donuts (blueberry glazed cake donuts for me, please, and apple fritters for Staci!) after each chemo appointment. Grief groups, both in person and online, normalize what isolation makes us question—that your reactions, your exhaustion, and even your conflicting emotions are human responses to extraordinary pain. As I often say about mental health: normalize, normalize, normalize that anticipatory grief is hard.

Staci: I joined an online support group because I have not been in a position to make time for another in-person meeting. At first, it felt good to join the group, a space for only patients with my specific diagnosis. Now, I encourage others as much as I can, but reading their stories feels scary to me. It creates a monster under my bed. So I do not spend as much time there anymore.

And then there are faith and spiritual communities. For some, they offer a sense of belonging when life feels fractured. They remind us of continuity—that love and meaning stretch beyond what we can see. For others, these spaces can be complicated. Rituals may offer comfort one moment and feel hollow the next. The prayers or scriptures that once soothed might now sting. This tension is part of the journey—grief breaks hearts, but it sometimes breaks belief systems too.

Faith as a Way of Holding

Bentina's faith carried her through this season in ways she is still coming to understand. Remember, she had to navigate her father's ALS diagnosis and make hard decisions as his power of attorney, which ultimately ended when he died during the COVID pandemic. He was taken to the hospital because he could no longer breathe on his own. The family said goodbye over FaceTime. Bentina, his health care power of attorney, made the decision alongside her mother to take him off the ventilator. Believing that her father was free from his broken body—reunited with loved ones—gave meaning to what might have otherwise felt unbearable.

Bentina says that within the African American community, faith often creates space for grief to be both mournful and celebratory. It allows sorrow and joy to exist side by side. Heaven is imagined not simply as absence but as freedom—release from pain, limitation, and suffering.

That belief did not erase grief. It did not quiet the loss. But it gave Bentina something to hold on to when the weight felt too heavy. Her experience opens a wider truth: Faith, in its broadest sense, is about relationship—to self, to others, and to something bigger than us. When grief shatters our sense of safety or meaning, spirituality can become a way of staying connected when certainty is no longer possible.

Spirituality can help us reweave a sense of belonging that transcends circumstances. In the anxious waiting of what's to come—and the uncertainty of how events will unfold—it's easy to feel isolated. Sometimes we pull away, hoping that distance will quiet the noise or make the pain less real. Yet faith calls us toward a different response. Scripture can remind us that the experience of anticipatory grief is not new; it has long been part of the human story of faith.

In the Garden of Gethsemane, as the weight of what awaited Him pressed heavily on His heart, Jesus said to His disciples, "My soul is overwhelmed with sorrow to the point of death. Stay here and keep watch with me" Matthew 26:38 (NIV). Faith does not remove the ache of what is coming; it gives us a way to bear it together. To "keep watch" is to remain tender to the reality of suffering, trusting that God is near in the waiting, in the uncertainty, and even in the sorrow that feels too heavy to name.

Rituals are particularly powerful because they give shape to what feels uncontainable. Lighting a candle at church, saying a name aloud, sharing a prayer before a meal—these small, repeated acts remind the body that connection endures, even across change or absence. Rituals externalize grief, allowing it to be expressed and processed.

But it's also important to name when the faith communities fall short. Sometimes, instead of sitting in the mystery with us, people rush to offer certainty—"They're in a better place" or "God has a plan." I can 100 percent tell you that the phrase "They're in a better place" sends me into lunar orbit. It's the wrong thing to say and minimizes the very real pain of loss. These phrases may be meant to comfort, but they often bypass the rawness of human emotion. In those moments, give yourself permission to protect your space. You don't owe anyone your spiritual energy while you're surviving the day-to-day weight of anticipatory grief.

If your faith has cracked, let it. Cracks are how the light gets back in. Many people find that over time, faith reemerges—softer, deeper, less about answers and more about connection. For some, this softening looks like letting go of rigid beliefs they once held tightly. Where faith used to be a checklist—pray hard enough, believe strongly enough, do the right things—it becomes something quieter. A whispered prayer in the car. A hand pressed to the heart before a medical update. A moment of stillness beside a hospital bed, asking for strength, even if you're not sure who you're asking.

For others, cracks in faith open the way to a more honest relationship with the divine. Instead of pretending to feel hopeful, they speak their fear plainly: "I'm angry," "I don't understand," or "Why her? Why him?"

This honesty often becomes its own kind of sacred because it is real.

Faith may also reemerge through small, unexpected moments—not through certainty but through resonance. A friend texts at the exact moment you feel like you're breaking. A nurse hums a familiar hymn while adjusting an IV line. Your loved one smiles in a way that feels like a benediction. You step outside after a long night, and the sunrise feels like a reminder that life still moves forward.

Some people discover that their faith shifts from doctrines to relationships—to the people who sit with them, bring meals, or simply refuse to let them walk this alone. Compassion becomes a form of prayer. Presence becomes a sanctuary.

And for many, the cracks create space for a gentler spirituality—one that doesn't demand certainty but invites curiosity: *What if faith is allowed to evolve? What if belief isn't something you hold perfectly but something that holds you? What if connection is enough?*

Faith after shattering is rarely the same as the faith you had before. But often, it's the faith that can hold your grief—and you—with more tenderness than the old one ever could.

STACI

My relationship with faith has been through the wringer. Thanks to the beautiful human I share life with, I'm now in a place where my faith and my values are aligned, even intertwined. The church has become a place of healing and peace for me, though I know that isn't true for everyone. In that space, I feel seen and cared for, and going to church helps recenter me on love and meaning.

Alongside that spiritual grounding, people have held me up. My friend Jake, a fellow cancer warrior, has been a steady guide from the very beginning. He offered support, let me ask every question, and shared practical advice, including the lidocaine-cream-and-plastic-wrap trick before your port is going to be accessed. He lets me ask him about my lab results and oral thrush, and we share infusion stories. We go to church together, so we also get to connect in person often. Honestly, I would not have made it this far without him; he is a literal angel. His generosity moved me to reach out to an acquaintance diagnosed with a different cancer a few weeks after me. I tried to pay his gift forward, and she and I have since become sisters. We check on each other and encourage each other regularly. Helping someone else has been life-giving.

Beyond individual friendships, I found a community online. I joined a support group specifically for people with lung cancer, a space that is both scary and normalizing. I'm not the only one going through this. The group helps temper self-pity, yet it also stirs my deepest fears, reminders of what could still happen.

And when words aren't enough, I go outside. The outdoors has become a place of solace. Perhaps there's something to the line, "From dust you came, and to dust you shall return." Maybe that's why I feel drawn to nature: to stand a little closer to where I began.

* * *

My relationship with faith has always been complicated. I grew up attending the Hungarian Congregational Church in Fairport Harbor, Ohio—a small town settled by Hungarian, Slovak, and Finnish immigrants in the early 1900s. My family was Hungarian, and so were the church services. That hour with my grandmother was painful. Imagine being five or six years old, sitting through a service where you couldn't understand a SINGLE word. That was my first experience with church.

As I got older, my generation witnessed the rise and fall of several prominent preachers who succumbed to the trappings of fame and money. I gave church a few more tries over the years, but I've ultimately settled into being *unchurched.* My husband's faith, however, is strong. He begins each day with either meditation or prayer.

I believe there is a higher power—as do most religions—but I don't think that power is vengeful. It's hard to see how religion has become so distorted in our country. I long for a soft place to land—a community rooted in compassion, where people genuinely care for one another, where helping neighbors and lifting the less fortunate are still sacred values. So far, I haven't found that place.

I also want to talk about community. Mine has grown smaller over the past year. Maybe that's because I've been carrying so much *hard* that the people I love no longer know what to say. Even my parents, who have been my anchors, are wrapped up in their own struggles. It's understandable but still painful. What has been remarkable, though, is the way Staci lets me talk about my dad, my mom, my stepmom, and my stepdad—even while she's carrying her own pain. I won't lie, I often feel guilty when I do this, but it isn't fair for me to opt her out of my life. She gets to make that choice, and she consistently chooses to show up for me. That kind of love—mutual, honest, imperfect—is what community looks like at its best.

Grief and faith both ask us to wrestle with mystery—to hold questions without clear answers and relationships that change shape over time. Community, in its truest form, meets us there. It doesn't demand certainty; it offers presence. As you think about your own journey, the reflections that follow are meant to help you explore where you find connection, what sustains you, and how you might begin to rebuild a sense of belonging—even in the midst of loss.

Journaling Exercise

- Who are my anchors right now? Identify one or two people who help you feel grounded. How can you reach out or allow them to show up for you?

- Where do I feel most connected? Is it in conversation, prayer, movement, nature, or creativity? How might you lean into that place of connection this week?

- How has my faith or worldview shifted during this season? What parts of your belief system have cracked—and what new light might be coming through?

- What small ritual can I create to honor connection? Choose one act—lighting a candle, journaling, sharing a memory—that helps you externalize what's inside.

Grief invites us to look at where we belong—and what belonging really means when life as we know it changes. Whether found in friendship, faith, ritual, or the natural world, connection gives shape to our suffering and lightens its weight. As we learn to stay connected, even in the face of uncertainty, we begin to rebuild a sense of home within ourselves. And it's from that inner home that we take our next steps. In the following chapter, we turn toward what it means to live in this in-between space: to hold love and loss side by side, to make room for both grief and meaning, and to move forward with the tenderness and courage this season requires.

Part IV

PREPARING FOR THE TRANSITION

Chapter 9

PRACTICAL AND EMOTIONAL

Grief has a way of pulling us between two worlds—one deeply practical and one entirely emotional. When someone we love is facing a serious illness or nearing the end of life, we're asked to think like caregivers, advocates, and project managers. It can feel like a lot. We are signing forms with shaky hands and making decisions while barely containing our tears. It is one of the hardest dualities of anticipatory grief: having to stay functional while feeling undone.

This chapter is about learning to balance the practical demands of care with the emotional realities of love, fear, and letting go. Because while medical choices, legal documents, and end-of-life planning are necessary, they are not separate from the emotional experience—they are emotional too. Every signature, every conversation, every choice is a declaration of care, even when it feels like shit.

Medical decisions during serious illness are rarely straightforward. There are treatment options to weigh, medications to manage, and appointments to coordinate. Each choice carries both logistical consequences and emotional weight. *Should we try another round of chemotherapy? When do we stop aggressive treatment and focus on comfort? What does "quality of life" really mean for our loved one—and for us?*

One of my clients, Carolyn A., shared with me, "The business of it all left me coping through a sort of sleepwalking or numbness. I didn't understand why this feeling was so pervasive. I understand it better now. I couldn't fall apart and manage hospital visits, family coming in, sitters, medication oversight, and all the rest. I felt guilty at night when I was too tired to cry."

These decisions are not about medicine alone. They're about values, identity, and love. As caregivers or family members, we want to respect the wishes of the person we love, but we also carry our own fears and hopes. It's common to feel torn between wanting to do everything possible and wanting them to have physical and emotional peace.

Staci: One thing that came up a few times was getting a second opinion, first from some friends and then from family. I have a high level of medical knowledge, but I am no doctor. What would I do with an alternate opinion, especially if it recommended a different treatment path? How would I decide between the two? So what finally landed for me was that I needed to be able to trust my medical team, especially my oncologist, and I knew without a doubt that I did. For me, a second opinion wouldn't be helpful; it would only cause more angst. And my family really heard that from me and respected it. A win for my bodily autonomy.

Staci's reflection highlights one of the core tensions of anticipatory grief and serious illness: the pull between wanting to explore every possible option and wanting peace. Her clarity about trusting her oncologist—and the relief that came once her family honored that—underscores how deeply personal these choices are. There is no universal right answer, only the one that preserves your sense of agency and steadiness in an already overwhelming time.

Serious illness brings a set of competing demands that can feel impossible to navigate. You may find yourself torn between wanting control and wanting to trust your medical team, between holding on to hope and confronting the realities of the prognosis, between honoring your own intuition and managing the expectations of well-meaning family members. You might swing between information overload and the need to stay informed, between protecting your autonomy and letting others support you, between shielding loved ones from worry and craving their comfort. Even the pace of decision-making becomes tense—the urge to act quickly colliding with the wisdom of giving choices time to settle. To balance these competing needs, try grounding each decision in two questions:

What matters most to them right now?

This centers on our person, not the disease. Their goals may change—from wanting more time to wanting more comfort or simply wanting a good day. Let those shifting values guide your choices.

What support do I need to make this decision well?

You do not have to carry this alone. Bring trusted family, clinicians, a family attorney, or spiritual advisors into the process. Ask doctors to explain not just what can be done but what should be done in alignment with your loved one's values. Ask the physician what they would do if this were their family member. I have found this very useful for caring for my parents.

Remember: Making medical decisions out of love doesn't mean doing everything possible to extend life—it means doing everything possible to honor life. This is an important distinction.

Conversations About Wishes, Dignity, and Comfort

Talking about the end of life feels like crossing an invisible boundary. It's uncomfortable, intimate, and sacred all at once. Many families delay these conversations, afraid they'll bring the sadness closer. But in truth, talking about wishes, dignity, and comfort is not giving up—it's showing up. Yeah, some of this really sucks.

When we invite our loved one to share what matters most to them—how they want to be cared for, what "comfort" means to them, what brings them peace—we are giving them a voice in how the rest of their story unfolds. These conversations are not morbid; they are deeply honoring. They say, "Your preferences, your values, and your humanity still matter. I'm here with you." You might begin gently, with open-ended questions:

- When you imagine the months ahead, what's most important to you?
- What makes a day feel meaningful or restful?
- Are there things you want us to know if you can't tell us later?

These conversations aren't one-time events; they evolve as the illness and emotions change. Some answers will shift. Some will deepen your person's resolve. Some will be surprising. Keeping that in mind, I've created a set of questions and topics to guide you—not as a checklist but as a pathway toward clarity, connection, and dignity.

Sometimes, dignity for your person looks like staying home. Other times, it's accepting help, rescheduling a treatment, shortening a visit, or listening to their favorite music while you sit together in silence. These conversations help you figure out what dignity looks like *today*—because it may not look the same tomorrow. Below are more questions and prompts that help keep those conversations open as the illness progresses.

Questions to Stay Emotionally Connected

Illness can create silence, distance, or withdrawal. These questions help soften that space:

- What's been weighing on you lately?
- What feels comforting right now? What feels overwhelming?
- How can I show up for you today in a way that feels supportive?

Gentle conversation starters:

- How is your heart today?
- What's one thing you want less of right now? What's one thing you want more of?

Questions About Evolving Needs and Preferences

Needs may shift weekly—sometimes daily. Revisit these often.

- What routines still feel good to you? Which ones feel too hard?
- What helps you feel safe when symptoms flare or emotions rise?
- Are there touchpoints—certain foods, smells, shows, music—that bring comfort?

Gentle conversation starters:

- Would you prefer visitors this week, or would quiet time be better for you?
- Do you want to talk through today's plan or just take it as it comes?

Questions for Navigating Hard Decisions

These keep clarity and compassion at the center when things get complex.

- If your energy is limited, what should we prioritize?
- What makes a medical intervention feel worth it to you?
- What would you want me to consider if a hard decision needs to be made?

Gentle conversation starters:

- If you ever can't speak for yourself, what values do you want to guide us?
- What does comfort care mean to you?

Comfort is not only physical—it's emotional and relational. It's knowing that you will respect your loved one's boundaries, hold their hand without fixing their feelings, and remember they are more than the diagnosis. I often think we get hung up on the "fixing" piece. Fixing gives us the illusion of control that we absolutely do not have, but for some, it provides purpose. Just make sure the need to fix does not conflict with your loved one's needs.

By the way, my husband, Tim, is the biggest fixer I have ever met. Most days, I love that about him. It's the way he checks in on my people, often calling out of the blue. It is also in the way that he has slowly taken over the daily chores at our house, taking on cleaning and cooking because my brain and body cannot do one more thing. It's how he shows love, and I am incredibly grateful for him. This allows me to spend my emotional capital on my people and traverse these difficult conversations with some energy left in my tank.

When we allow these conversations to happen, we lessen the burden later—for ourselves and for others. Clarity brings peace. It means that when decisions need to be made, love can guide us instead of fear and panic.

STACI

There was a night early on in my treatment when Amy, Greg, and I were sitting in our TV room. I was completely worn down from the chemo, the kind of exhaustion that sinks into your bones. I was lying on the couch, and they were sitting on the floor, almost as if they were holding vigil for anything I needed. I asked both if I could ask a tricky question. I wanted to know if they could and wanted to be the ones responsible for respecting my wishes at the end of my life. I assume the end will be a struggle for the people who love me, and I want them to let me go rather than intervene. I want nature to take its course once I stop treatment. It felt important to talk about it early, in case either of them did not want that burden, which I would absolutely understand.

They didn't hesitate. They immediately said yes; they knew what I wanted and were willing to honor it.

Greg and I have also talked about where I want to be at the end of my life. If I could script it, I'd be staring out at the ocean.

But since dying in someone's Airbnb feels awkward at best, we had to talk about reality. I assumed Greg wouldn't want me to die in our home. I know I wouldn't want to continue living in a house after he died in it. But he surprised me. He said that is precisely what he wants: for me to be home.

Conversations like these are never easy, but they anchor us to the truth of what matters most, and now, as we return to this chapter, they remind us why planning, even when uncomfortable, is an act of love.

Remember: Clear is kind. Have the hard conversations.

Advance Care Planning: Love in Action

Advance care planning is one of the most practical and compassionate steps you can take during an illness. It transforms anxiety about the unknown into a shared plan that reflects your loved one's values. This process typically includes:

- **Advance directives:** Documents that specify medical wishes and designate a health care proxy.
- **Living will:** A statement outlining what kinds of interventions are wanted (or not wanted) if the person can't communicate.
- **Durable power of attorney for health care:** The person legally chosen to make decisions on your loved one's behalf.
- **Five wishes or values-based plans:** Written tools that address not just treatment but also personal and spiritual priorities (e.g., "I want soft music playing," "I want my pet nearby," "I want my family to know I forgive them.").

You met Dr. Bill Walker in an earlier chapter. When I asked him how he and his family approached this kind of planning, he told me, "In the case of my wife, we built what we call the *red file* together and made a pact that whoever survives will ensure those wishes are carried out. We started building that file shortly after I got my first 'real job.' Our kids have always known it exists, and now that they're in their late twenties, we're intentionally planning a sit-down with them, along with our lawyer and financial advisor, so that they can understand the general outline. Anything tangible we leave behind is accounted for in the red folder."

Dr. Walker credits much of this organization to his financial advisor, a man named Jim. "I can only wish I had known how to do any of the hard stuff," he said. "And then, just like magic, a guy named Jim was put in my life." I love that Bill had no problem asking for help. People do these hard things for a living; it's just about finding one that makes sense for you.

As a counselor, I am not an expert in these things, but I do know that this is not something to navigate alone. Please make sure you are working with a reputable family attorney to get all this right. It is worth the investment. If you are the one initiating these conversations, start by framing them in love: "I want to make sure we're honoring what matters most to you—not just medically but emotionally and spiritually."

Advance care planning is not about control—it's about care. It gives everyone involved a shared language for dignity. It helps prevent conflict and guilt later, when emotions are high and clarity is hard to find. Even when it feels overwhelming, this work is an act of devotion.

There will be moments when you're filling out forms, scheduling hospice consultations, or sorting medications, and the tears come unexpectedly. You might feel guilty for crying, as if there's no time for emotion amid the logistics. But this, too, is grief—the intersection of duty and love. Allow yourself to feel. Each form signed, each decision made, each conversation had is an expression of your love. You are not just managing tasks—you are building a bridge of care for someone you love. Please don't forget to take care of yourself, even if it's just a deep breath or a five-minute break.

When possible, create rituals of rest and meaning around the process. After a difficult appointment, take a walk, listen to music, call someone who understands, or scream out loud to break the tension. These small pauses help integrate the emotional and the pragmatic, keeping your heart from becoming buried under the mounds of responsibility.

Journaling Exercise: Leading with Love

- What has been the hardest decision I have faced so far?

- What fears do I have about talking openly about end-of-life care?

- What matters most to my loved one—and how do I know?

- What small act could make this process feel more loving and less clinical?

Grief will always be both practical and emotional—both planning and feeling, both action and ache. Balancing these worlds doesn't make the experience less painful, but it can make it more meaningful.

STACI

I've always been oddly comfortable with death. I even explored the idea of becoming a death doula, and for years, I had this odd feeling that I would die at sixty-six. Maybe that will still be true, but this diagnosis suggests I may have been wrong. Long before this stupid cancer, I talked and even joked about death. I know that can put people off; my mom refuses to entertain those conversations, my partner has gradually come around, and most of my close friends have adapted.

Because of that history, I believe it's important to get comfortable with death, and I recognize I've had an unusual advantage: I've spent my career talking about hard things. A few weeks ago, during the icebreaker at a work meeting for long-term planning, we were asked to pair up and share what would be true about our lives in twelve years. I simply said, "I'll be dead." Maybe that sounded blunt, but cancer has made me less willing to prioritize other people's comfort, about my illness or anything else, over honesty.

For me, planning is an act of love. Only seventeen weeks (about four months) into this cancer, I've already started making my wishes clear:

- *I've asked my favorite badass minister to preach at my funeral.*
- *I've chosen a burial spot.*
- *I made my partner get long-term care insurance.*
- *I've begun a list of funeral details: sunflowers and magnolias everywhere, bright colors and protest T-shirts, a few poems and songs, a tasteful reception at the church, and an after-party at our favorite restaurant.*

That clarity extends to our everyday life. I've started clearing out my things. My partner teases me about all my "stuff," and he's not wrong; my closet is jam-packed, and there's even overflow in the guest bathtub. It feels good to purge—to let a friend "shop" my closet and to let go of books I'll never read again.

I can't emphasize this enough: Make the plans. Write a will. Choose who will make medical decisions on your behalf. I even snagged a spot in the new columbarium at Oakland Cemetery today.

I've also started saying "I love you" so often that it makes people a little uncomfortable, and I'm okay with that. When mortality is in the room, love deserves to be louder.

As for regret, I know it often surfaces when we face death. I don't live there much. Of course, there are things I wish I'd done differently, but the grass on the other side is rarely as green as we imagine. I'm focusing on apologies I need to make and on making peace with mistakes that may have hurt others. I'm also wrestling with forgiveness, especially regarding my biological mother. We haven't spoken since 1988, and she smoked around me for the first fifteen years of my life; there's a lot to unpack. I'm at peace, even if I'm not yet at forgiveness. If you haven't read The Midnight Library, *I recommend it for a thoughtful lens on regret.*

People keep asking about a bucket list. I don't have one. The big dreams, like going to Paris, I've already done. What I'm working on now is reimagining joy: finding smaller, more present ways it can show up for me, even if my capacity is different from what it used to be.

* * *

The paperwork for all my parents was completed years ago, with a few modifications along the way as relationships and circumstances evolved. Each set of parents created a trust—a legal tool that helps loved ones inherit assets more quickly and privately (or as my parents like to joke, "if there's anything left") while avoiding the lengthy and often expensive probate process. A trust allows them to control exactly how and when wealth is passed down, set conditions for distributions, and ensure that their financial and health care wishes are honored.

The only part we haven't discussed in detail is what type of service they would like after they've passed, though all of them have chosen cremation. The process so far has been remarkably straightforward—almost surprisingly so—and, to my relief, not particularly emotional. I think that's because this kind of preparation is an act of love disguised as logistics. It may seem practical on the surface, but it carries profound emotional generosity underneath. By making these decisions ahead of time, my parents have given me one of the greatest gifts imaginable: the ability to grieve without being weighed down by paperwork, confusion, or the fear of making the wrong choice. When the time comes, I can focus on being there and remembering them.

STACI

When Meagan and I talked to David—remember, he's the friend living with ALS—one of the things that struck me most was how much of his time is spent planning for the end of his life. When you don't have a partner to help shoulder those decisions, everything becomes more complicated. He had toured a few senior living communities, hoping to find a place that felt safe and supportive, but something about each one felt off. Now, he's wrestling with the question of how his care will be managed when he can no longer meet his own needs. It's a heavy, lonely calculus, one that reveals just how much vulnerability and courage this season demands.

Journaling Exercise

The Gift of Preparation

- What decisions or conversations could you begin now that might ease the burden for those you love later? What would it feel like to see that preparation as a gift—not a chore?

Facing the Uncomfortable

- What makes it difficult to talk about end-of-life plans or services with your loved ones? Are there fears, family dynamics, or emotions that get in the way?

Honoring Their Wishes

- Have you talked with your loved ones about what kind of service, celebration, or remembrance feels meaningful to them—or to you? What would it look like to make those wishes part of your shared story rather than a future task?

Relief and Readiness

- How might planning ahead free emotional space for grief, healing, and reflection when the time comes?

Preparation doesn't erase grief, but it creates room for it. When the logistical pieces are handled, our hearts have more space to feel, remember, and honor. Conversations about end-of-life care, finances, and wishes can feel uncomfortable.

Still, they are, at their core, conversations about love—about wanting to protect one another from chaos and confusion in moments already heavy with emotion. Planning is not a denial of death; it's an embrace of life's whole arc. When we make peace with these details now, we make space later for what truly matters—presence, memory, and connection.

Chapter 11

WHEN THE TIME COMES

Once the paperwork is finished and the decisions are made, there's often a quiet pause—a moment when the practical work is complete but the emotional work is just beginning. Preparing the heart is a different kind of task. It's not about signatures or checklists; it's about softening into the reality that loss is coming and learning how to hold that truth without letting it consume you.

Emotional readiness doesn't mean detachment. It means developing the capacity to stay present even when the thought of saying goodbye makes your chest tighten. It's giving yourself permission to feel *everything*—sadness, fear, gratitude, even relief—without judging any of it. These emotions are not signs of weakness; they're evidence of love stretching itself around something too big to control.

Preparing the heart often begins with honesty. You may notice small internal whispers that say, *I can't imagine life without them* or *I'm not ready.* Those thoughts are invitations, not failures. They invite you to acknowledge what is real—the tenderness of anticipation, the ache of uncertainty—and to practice compassion toward yourself in the middle of all of it.

This kind of readiness also asks for presence. Rather than rushing to stay busy or distracted, try slowing down. Sit with your loved one a little longer, linger over a shared memory, or say the things that have been left unsaid. If an apology is needed, say it. If you haven't told them you love them, say it. Say anything you need now so you don't regret it later. These small moments of connection become the threads you'll hold on to later.

As you transition and begin to accept the loss, it can help to name what you fear most about their death—and to notice what, if anything, brings a sense of peace. As we discussed previously, some people find grounding in faith or ritual, others in nature, movement, or stillness. There's no single way to prepare emotionally for loss because there's no single way to love.

Ultimately, preparing the heart is about weaving resilience and tenderness together. It's about trusting that when the time comes, you'll have what you need—not because you've planned every detail but because you've practiced being honest with yourself and your loved one. The goal isn't to be ready for the loss—it's to be *real* in the face of it.

What It Means to Be Present at the End

Being present at the end of a loved one's life is one of the most profound acts of love we can offer as human beings. Presence doesn't require the perfect words or a grand gesture—it simply asks that we *stay*. To sit beside someone as they take their final breaths is to hold space for both the mystery of life and the reality of death. It may mean listening to their stories one last time, holding their hand in silence, or comforting them as they struggle with their reality. In these moments, your calm becomes their comfort. Calm presence allows us to witness the transition between life and death—to say, "You are not alone."

It's not easy. When we choose to stay, even in the face of our own fear or sadness, we remind ourselves that showing up—heart open—is sometimes the most healing thing we can do.

Staci here. One of the things I watched this year was Dying for Sex. *If you're facing the death of a loved one, I genuinely recommend it. It's a beautiful, honest series that captures the end of life without sugarcoating the hard parts. What stood out to me is how clearly it explains things most people don't know, like what a "surge" is. When someone is dying, that sudden burst of energy isn't an improvement; it's the body's final rally. Or how, in the last days, your loved one will likely stop eating and start sleeping most of the day. It's not them giving up. It's their body preparing for the transition.*

Knowing those things doesn't make grief easier, but it does help you plan for what's coming. It forces you to think about how you want to spend the time you still have, what conversations matter, what moments you want to savor, and what you can let go of. It also helps you understand that there won't magically be space at the end for long, movie-style goodbyes.

Being present at the end of life is one of the most profound acts of love—and yet, for many, it's also one of the most frightening. The thought of watching someone you love die can stir deep fear, helplessness, or even panic. For some, it awakens old wounds—memories of previous losses or unresolved trauma that resurface in moments of vulnerability. Others find that medical environments themselves make presence more complicated. Hospitals and hospice rooms, though filled with care, can feel sterile, with the hum of machines and the rhythm of staff moving from one patient to another. It's easy to feel small in those spaces, like your love is competing with time, protocols, and beeping monitors.

These barriers are real and human. They don't mean you're weak or unloving; they mean you're *feeling*. The emotional discomfort we experience around dying often mirrors how our culture avoids it—we are not taught how to sit with endings. We try to control, fix, or soften what is inherently uncontrollable. Sometimes, we hide behind busyness or medical details because it's easier than facing the reality of loss head-on. But presence doesn't ask for perfection. It asks for courage—the willingness to stay, to breathe, and to bear witness even when it hurts.

Different forms of presence:

- **Physical:** Sitting bedside, holding a hand, offering comfort.
- **Emotional:** Remaining grounded ("I'm here. Tell me what's coming up for you"), being honest without overwhelming your person ("I feel scared too, but we're facing this together") even as fear or anticipatory sorrow surge.
- **Spiritual:** Creating ritual, prayer, or stillness that gives meaning to the moment.

Presence is not about *doing*; it's about *being*. You don't have to know the right words or provide constant reassurance. It might look like adjusting a pillow, brushing hair from a forehead, or whispering, "I'm here." These small acts matter because they remind both of you that love is still alive in the room—even as the body begins to let go.

Reframing Presence

When fear rises, it helps to reframe what it means to be there. Instead of thinking, *I need to make this better,* try reminding yourself, *I am not here to fix it. I am here to honor my loved one.*

You cannot stop what is happening, but you can choose how you will meet it. Honoring means respecting the sacred threshold between life and death—allowing it to unfold without trying to force it into something tidy or comfortable. It means focusing on the human connection rather than the medical process.

From a clinical perspective, mindfulness and breath awareness can help anchor you in those moments. Slow, intentional breathing regulates your nervous system, keeping you from slipping into panic or emotional dissociation. When your mind races or your body tenses, return to your breath. Feel your feet on the floor, your hand on theirs, the air moving in and out of your lungs. That rhythm—steady and grounding—reminds you that you are alive, connected, and safe enough to stay.

It also makes me sad to know that breath is not something Staci can do to anchor herself. Her lungs are where her disease lives, and focusing there is a distraction at best and a trigger at worst. We will have to find another way.

Sometimes, presence also means allowing yourself to step out for a moment. Taking breaks doesn't mean you've failed; it means you're human. A brief walk down the hallway, a few minutes by a window, or a moment of prayer or journaling can help you reregulate before returning to the bedside. Presence is a practice of pacing yourself—staying close enough to offer love while also tending to your own emotional limits.

Ultimately, presence at the end is an act of sacred witnessing. You are saying, "I see you. I love you. You are not alone." It's the purest form of compassion—not fixing, not saving, but accompanying. In the quiet of that kind of presence, healing happens—not of the body but of the heart.

Journaling Exercise

- What does it mean for me to show up fully—even as I prepare for goodbye? Consider how you can remain emotionally present, even when it hurts to watch someone decline. What does "showing up" look like for you—listening, comforting, laughing, holding, remembering—and how might it shift as your loved one's needs change?

- What parts of me want to turn away, and what are they protecting? Reflect on the moments you feel yourself pulling back—becoming busy, distracted, or numb. What fear, memory, or pain are those parts trying to protect you from? How might you gently thank them for their effort while still staying connected?

- How can I balance being present with taking care of my own heart? Being near illness and loss takes a toll. What helps you refill emotionally—time alone, prayer, nature, talking with a trusted friend or counselor?

- What conversations or moments still feel unfinished? Think about words you still want to say, questions you want to ask, or memories you want to share. What might it look like to begin those now—not to rush closure but to create peace and understanding for both of you?

- What will "showing up fully" mean when they are gone? Grief doesn't end with death. How might you carry forward what you learned from them—their values, humor, or love—as a way of continuing connection and honoring their legacy?

- How can I offer compassion to myself in the moments I can't bear to stay? There will be times you need space. When that happens, what words or actions could remind you that stepping away isn't failure—it's part of surviving an unbearable reality?

The Threshold: From Anticipation to After

I am standing on the threshold of death, knowing it will happen "sometime." Will it be my mom, my stepdad, my dad, my stepmom, my husband, Staci, Cooper, or someone else I have not anticipated? As I write this chapter, death has not yet shown up. Still, I find myself *rehearsing* the phone call I imagine will come from the other parent or the hospital—when the time arrives. My thoughts often wander to what will happen if my dad dies at home and my stepmom, too cognitively impaired to help, does nothing. There are days I close my eyes and can picture Staci's memorial service.

In my gallows humor, I call this my *exposure therapy*—exposing myself to the things that cause me anxiety so that I might no longer be as anxious. Yes, this is a real type of therapy that works for clients with obsessive-compulsive disorder, an extreme form of anxiety—but I digress.

And while I still am afraid, it is no longer as all-encompassing as it was six or nine months ago. I have learned to take better care of myself, stay anchored in the here and now, and spend far more time with the people I genuinely care about. And I'm starting to see those choices show up in real, tangible ways.

Today was hard. This summer, Tim spent hours tracking down Johnny G. during reunion planning. Why did he take the extra time? Johnny was one of the first friends Tim made when he moved to Chapel Hill at fourteen, leaving behind Montclair, New Jersey, and starting over in a new state.

Johnny didn't have an email address or a cell phone, so Tim eventually reached him on his landline. The phone number was originally his parents' and was the only contact information Tim had from back in high school. Johnny showed up to the reunion, and Tim got to see him—neither of them knowing he was sick.

Last week, they talked on the phone, and Tim said goodbye—something I'm not sure he would have done a decade ago in the same way. He has stopped fighting his feelings and his need to be in control and has allowed himself to grieve. Johnny's sister told Tim his passing would be quick, and it was.

I'm sure Tim has thought about his own mortality. I think about it too. But today, I am choosing to love my husband fiercely—to make a meal that nourishes him and hold him tight. Those are the only things I can control. He doesn't need fixing; he needs time to grieve. One day, I will need the same thing, and if he is here, I know he will show up for me.

Grief is a quiet rehearsal for love—the way it asks us to stay present, even as we sense the edges of loss forming. I am learning that preparation for death is not about bracing for impact but about softening into what matters most. It is about tending to life while we still have it: cooking the meal, making the call, saying "I love you" when words feel small but necessary. Anticipatory grief has taught me that I cannot control when or how death comes, but I can choose how I meet it—with tenderness, honesty, and the courage to remain open, even when my heart wants to break.

The instant of death is when you must step over the threshold, a quiet crossing point where anticipatory grief gives way to conventional grief. For days, months, or even years, your body and mind have been preparing for this moment, bracing for its arrival. And then, suddenly, it happens. Time feels strange here—it both stands still and rushes forward. The air changes, the room feels different, and you know, without anyone having to say it, that something sacred has occurred. The anticipation that once filled every breath dissolves, replaced by a heavy stillness. This is the moment when your waiting ends and your mourning begins. Your loved one has died.

In the minutes and hours that follow, you might feel a mix of emotions that seem to contradict each other—disbelief, relief, guilt, numbness, even calm. The nervous system, long attuned to vigilance, doesn't know where to go next. Many describe this period as both surreal and grounding, as if part of you is watching life continue while another part is still sitting by the bedside. The brain, which has lived for so long in the rhythm of "what if," now must learn to live with "what is."

The threshold is not a single moment but a passage. It takes time for the heart, the body, and the mind to catch up to one another. Crossing this boundary gently means allowing yourself to feel the full weight of both love and loss—not pushing it away but letting it move through you. In this space, grief stops being anticipatory and becomes lived. It's the beginning of learning how to carry on with your life in your loved one's absence. It is also a reminder that this relationship is deeply ingrained in your body and mind. Both will anticipate the return of your loved one for some period of time. We are wired for this connection, which is part of why grief can feel so painful.

Counselor's Note: The Coexistence of Relief and Sorrow

It's common to feel relief when a loved one's suffering ends—and just as common to feel guilty for that relief. You might think, *What kind of person feels lighter after someone dies?* But relief doesn't mean you wished for their death. It means your body and mind are recognizing that the long season of uncertainty, vigilance, and emotional strain has come to an end. The release you feel comes from the exhaustion of loving someone through decline.

Sorrow and relief can—and often do—coexist. They are not opposing emotions but two sides of the same experience. One honors the depth of your attachment; the other acknowledges the toll of prolonged caregiving and anticipatory grief. Feeling relief does not diminish the love you carry. In fact, it can reflect just how deeply you've been present.

When clients tell me they feel "wrong" for feeling both, I remind them that the nervous system can only stay on high alert for so long. When death comes, the body sometimes exhales before the heart catches up. That exhale—that tiny flicker of peace—is a physiological truth, not a moral failure.

The work of grief is learning to hold these contradictions without shame. Relief does not erase sorrow; sorrow does not invalidate relief. Both are valid. Both are human. Allowing them to coexist is how healing begins—not by choosing one emotion over another but by making space for the whole, complicated truth of love and loss.

In addition to relief and sorrow, you may experience other emotions that are often unpredictable. Many people describe a sense of numbness or disbelief, a feeling that it's not real. This shock is the mind's way of protecting the heart—creating temporary distance from a reality too painful to absorb all at once. Others experience guilt for feeling relief or calm, as if the easing of tension or suffering somehow betrays their love. It doesn't. Still others notice an unexpected surge of energy or busyness, diving into arrangements and family logistics as a way to stay functional. This burst of activity often masks the deeper undercurrent of grief, buying time until the emotions catch up. None of these responses are wrong. They are simply the body and mind finding ways to navigate the shock of transition—the threshold between holding on and letting go.

Journaling Exercise: Holding Relief and Sorrow Together

- Name what you feel: When you think about your loved one's death or decline, what emotions come first? Write them down without editing or organizing them. Notice if relief shows up alongside sadness, gratitude, or even emptiness. Use the feelings wheel to help with this response.

- Give each emotion a voice: If your relief could speak, what would it say? What about your sorrow? Let each emotion express itself fully. There is no need to choose between them—all of them deserve space and understanding.

- Release the guilt: What stories have you told yourself about what it *means* to feel relief? Are those stories true, or are they rooted in shame, fear of judgment, or a "should"? How might you reframe relief as a sign of endurance, compassion, or closure rather than wrongdoing?

- Integrate the truth: Grief is not a single feeling but a collection of contradictions. How can you honor both your love and your exhaustion, your sorrow and your peace without trying to resolve them?

Grief rarely moves in straight lines. It is full of surprises and feelings we don't expect to coexist. Relief and sorrow, love and exhaustion, peace and pain—they all belong to the same emotional landscape. The goal is not to sort or silence them but to allow them to sit side by side without judgment. In our world that rewards busyness and instant recovery from grief, we have not been taught to sit with these feelings for any length of time.

I promise you the best way forward is through, giving grief all the attention it deserves. If you don't do that, your body will punish you. If you don't believe me, read *The Body Keeps the Score*. I referenced it earlier in the book. If you were married for twenty years and your spouse died, could you recover in a week or two? If your best friend of thirty years died, could you bounce back in a week? I write these questions to highlight the absurdity of the notion that grief is a brief stop on our journey. In the end, grief asks for honesty more than order.

As the sharpness of immediate grief begins to settle, another question emerges: *What now?* When the waiting ends and the world feels too quiet, rituals and acts of meaning become anchors in the aftermath. They give the heart something to do when there are no more tasks left to complete. Rituals—whether private or shared—help translate what feels unspeakable into something visible and sacred. They remind us that love does not end when life does; it simply changes form. Moving from relief and sorrow into ritual is not about finding closure—it's about finding continuity, a way to keep love present even in the absence of the person who carried it.

The Quiet After

There is a stillness that follows the storm—not empty but sacred. When the time comes, love remains. The work of anticipatory grief shifts from holding on to learning how to move forward. The next chapter begins not with forgetting but with remembering differently. What once was preparation now becomes the practice of living in the aftermath—heart open, feet on new ground.

CHAPTER 12

FROM ANTICIPATORY TO ACTIVE GRIEF

When death arrives, the world changes shape. The familiar rhythms of care and anticipation are replaced by stillness, absence, and the ache of finality.

Rituals for After the Death

Rituals help us bridge the space between what was and what is—they remind our bodies and hearts that love does not end; it only changes form. Not all of these will resonate with you, and that's okay. Find one or two that do or work on finding a ritual that makes sense for you based on family or cultural norms.

- **The first quiet moment:** After the initial shock, take a breath. Sit in silence—in a chair, in the car, or by their bedside—and allow the reality to land gently. Whisper their name. Offer a simple sentence of gratitude: "Thank you for loving me" or "Thank you for letting me love you."
- **The candle ritual:** Light a candle each evening for the first week or month after their passing. As the flame

flickers, say a short prayer, memory, or hope for peace. The candle becomes a symbol of ongoing connection—a reminder that their light remains. And you now hold part of that light within you.

- **Creating a memory space:** Choose a small corner in your home for photographs, letters, or a few cherished objects. This space doesn't have to be permanent—it simply gives your grief a place to go. Visit it when you need to remember, talk, or weep.
- **The letter you didn't get to send:** Write a letter to your loved one. Include what you didn't say, what you wish they knew, and what you are carrying forward. Some people place it near their loved one's urn or grave; others burn or bury it as an act of release.
- **The shared story:** Tell a story about them—even a small, ordinary one—to someone who never met them. Each retelling keeps them alive in a new way. Grief becomes less lonely when memories are openly talked about.
- **The body's return to rhythm:** After a loss, even simple acts like eating, walking, or showering can feel impossible. Choose one gentle daily ritual—morning tea, stretching, or stepping outside to feel the sun—to remind your body that life continues.
- **Annual remembrances:** Mark anniversaries, birthdays, or meaningful dates with intention. Visit their favorite place, make their favorite meal, or play a song that reminds you of them. Rituals of remembrance offer continuity—the ability to honor without being trapped by pain.
- **The legacy ritual:** Ask yourself, *How do I carry their love forward?* Perhaps through doing an act of kindness in

their name, mentoring someone, or supporting a cause they cared about. The goal is not to replace them but to continue the story or the work they invested in.

- **The ritual of rest:** Grief is exhausting. Allow yourself to rest. Sleep is one of the most important things we can do to support our emotional and physical health. Light a candle before bed, take a deep breath, and say aloud, "It is safe to rest. They are at peace, and I can rest too."
- **The return to life:** Eventually, you will laugh again, plan again, and hope again. This, too, is a ritual—the living continuation of their love through you. Returning to life is an integral part of the grieving process. Your life may look different now, and that is okay.

In time, the rituals you choose will soften into rhythm. What begins as deliberate remembrance becomes part of the fabric of daily life—a photo you look at each day, a song that feels like a quiet hello. Grief is not something to complete but something to carry, and these rituals teach us how to do it. They remind us that love does not vanish when the body is gone; it transforms, becoming presence rather than touch, memory rather than conversation. The work now is learning how to live alongside what remains—to let love guide the way forward, one breath, one small act of remembrance at a time.

Importance of Meaning-Making

In the days and weeks following death, the work of meaning-making becomes vital. It is the process by which we reconstruct coherence and significance in the aftermath of death, thereby fostering adaptation and emotional healing. Research shows that meaning-making is a key factor in adapting to bereavement, the fancy word for loss.

Studies demonstrate that individuals who can find meaning—whether through spiritual frameworks, connection to others, or new life purpose—experience fewer symptoms of prolonged or complicated grief. For instance, Davis and colleagues found that bereaved individuals who were able to make sense of their loss and see benefits from it had significantly lower levels of distress and depression.[41] Later research by Lichtenthal and Neimeyer confirmed that difficulties in meaning reconstruction were strongly associated with prolonged grief and poorer mental health outcomes.[42] Meaning-centered grief therapy, developed by Neimeyer and colleagues, has since shown that intentionally exploring and reconstructing meaning after loss can help restore a sense of purpose, identity, and connection.

Meaning-making does not erase pain. It allows grief to evolve from *Why did this happen?* to *How will I live now?* Through this process, the person left behind often discovers ways to carry forward the essence of the person who died—their values, their humor, their love—as part of their own ongoing story. In doing so, meaning-making becomes a bridge between grief and growth, helping us live with both loss and life at once.

Journaling Exercise: Making Meaning After Loss

- How has this loss changed the story I tell about myself and my life? Consider how your sense of identity, purpose, or worldview has shifted since the death.

- What beliefs, values, or lessons from my loved one continue to guide me? Reflect on how their presence still shapes your choices or how you show up in the world.

- What have I learned about love, connection, or resilience through this experience? Grief often deepens our understanding of what truly matters. What wisdom has it revealed?

- Where do I find moments of meaning or peace, even briefly? Think about rituals, relationships, or quiet practices that help you stay connected to life.

- How can I carry forward my loved one's legacy in a way that feels authentic? Meaning-making is not about moving on—it's about integrating love into the life that continues.

CLOSING REFLECTION

Anticipatory grief changes us. It strips away illusions of control, softens edges we didn't know we had, and opens spaces inside us where love and loss coexist. When I began writing this book, I thought I was capturing one story—mine and Staci's—but what I discovered was a tapestry of stories: of friends, clients, family members, and readers who, in their own ways, have stood on the threshold of loss and dared to stay present.

If you've made it to this point, I hope that you feel less alone. That you've found language for what once felt unspeakable. That you've begun to see anticipatory grief not as something to fix but as something to honor—proof of how deeply you love. I also hope you feel a sense of companionship—that in these pages, you've found words for what you may have struggled to name. I hope you've discovered tools to help you tend to your own anticipatory grief: reflection questions that guide, practices that ground, and stories that remind you that healing is not a single moment of arrival but an ongoing act of courage.

The truth is there is no "getting over" loss. There is only learning to live alongside it, to let it shape you without defining you. You will still laugh. You will still find moments of beauty, of connection, of unexpected peace. You will keep becoming.

As you move forward, may you grant yourself permission to be both broken and whole, hopeful and hurting, grateful and grieving—sometimes all in the same breath. Let your story continue to unfold, not despite your loss but through it.

And when the world feels heavy again, return to the small rituals that ground you—a walk outside, a quiet cup of tea, a deep breath that reminds you you're still here—because healing is not a destination. It's a way of traveling—slowly, gently, one honest moment at a time.

ACKNOWLEDGMENTS

This book would not exist without the generosity, courage, and honesty of the people who allowed us into some of the most tender seasons of their lives. We are deeply grateful to **David Jernigan**, **Bentina Chisholm Terry**, and **Dr. Bill Walker** for trusting us with their stories.

David, your willingness to speak openly about vulnerability, planning, and the quiet courage it takes to face the unknown gave this book a grounding truth. You reminded us that strength is not found in avoiding hard conversations but in leaning into them with clarity and intention.

Bentina, your story is a testament to the power of love, faith, and family. The way you held both grief and hope at the same time offered us—and our readers—a beautiful example of how meaning can emerge even in the most painful seasons. Your voice carries wisdom that will resonate with so many.

Dr. Walker, your perspective brought both professional insight and human warmth to these pages. Your reflections helped bridge the clinical and the personal, reminding us that behind every diagnosis, plan, or treatment is a deeply human story.

To each of you: Thank you for your openness, trust, and willingness to let your experiences become a source of comfort and guidance for others. Your stories are not just part of this book—they are part of its heart.

Special thanks to our founding members who invested in us and the vision for this book:

Andrea Dill
Tawnya Freund
Julie O'Brien
Tameka Rish
Tamara Stevens
Alan and Rebecca Thomas
Joellen Wooten

Special thanks to our sustaining members for supporting this book:

Amy Kennedy
Lynn and Candace Fowler
Stuart and Becky Hoff
Yvette Connor

Additional thanks to:

Damon Elmore, Ashley Byrd, Charisse Williams, Kath Conver, Whitney Deal, Amanda Sapp, Dan Gordon, Jody Greenwood, Ariel Fristoe, Julia Houston, Ann Duffy, Sandi Lodge, Kathie Anderson, Matthew Holder, Lauri Strauss, Nancy Hohmann, Anne Henn, Kevin Click, Brigitte Peck, Karri Sauer, Shannon Livingston, Carroll Sterne, Daniel Ostick, Dee LaMay, Becca Sherrill, Beth Mattern, Jeff Shamis, Frances Justice, Melinda Kelleher, Jen Slipakoff, Jill Surrency Roark, Michael Cabe, Lindesy Chapman, Laura Guerin, Leeann Jones, Kristina Koldoff Christy, Julie Kohn, Patricia Lassiter, Jennifer Saliers, Lisa Keyes, Ann Carol Pence, Aimee Cunningham, Melinda Holladay, Alicia Jones, Rachel Ziglar, Betsy Liley, Jen Cox,

Shannon Cho, Lisa Dwyer, Phil Smith, Monique Honaman, Rissa Reddan, Jeff Teague, Kelly Aissen, Constance Callahan, Shelby KM, Cheryl Molenaar, Arefe Moosajee Cassoobhoy, Ivette Sisniega, Angela Blagdon, Tiffany Layden, Aaron Swain, Nellie Sullivan, Janice Barrocas, Tom Subak.

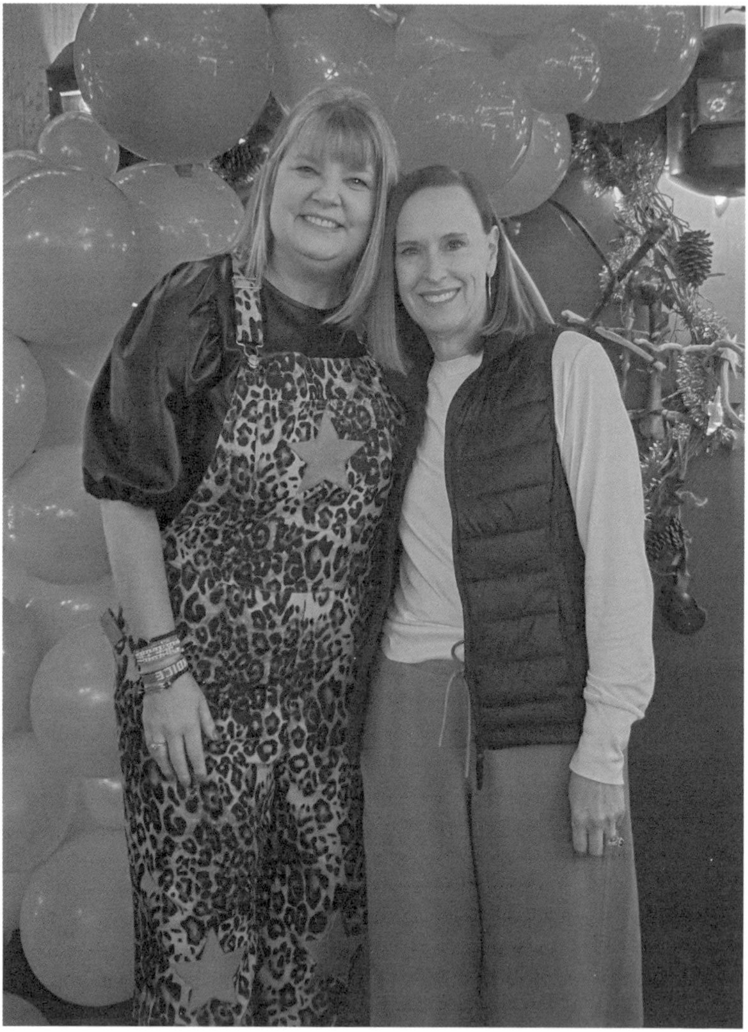

RESOURCES

Immediate Crisis Support

- **988 Suicide & Crisis Lifeline:** Call or text 988 anytime in the US for free, confidential support.
- **911:** For life-threatening emergencies.
- **NAMI Helpline:** 1-800-950-NAMI (6264)

National Alliance on Mental Health https://www.nami.org/

Mental Health America https://mhanational.org/

The Mental Health Coalition https://www.thementalhealthcoalition.org/

National Institute of Mental Health https://www.nimh.nih.gov/

Anxiety & Depression Association of America https://adaa.org/

Black Emotional and Mental Health Collective https://beam.community/

American Foundation for Suicide Prevention https://afsp.org/

Finding a Therapist

Psychology Today https://www.psychologytoday.com/us

Headway https://care.headway.co/intake/care-type?flow=growth&lat=34.02343&lon=-84.61549&state=georgia

Therapy Tribe https://www.therapytribe.com/therapist/united-states/

Alma https://secure.helloalma.com/providers-landing/

Therapy for Black Girls https://therapyforblackgirls.com/

Black Female Therapists https://blackfemaletherapists.com/

Zencare https://zencare.co/

National Register of Health Service Psychologists https://www.findapsychologist.org/cities/

Psychologist Locator https://locator.apa.org/

FindTreatment.gov https://findtreatment.gov/

The Trevor Project https://www.thetrevorproject.org/

National Queer & Trans Therapists of Color Network https://nqttcn.com/

Black Virtual Wellness Directory https://wellness.beam.community/

VA Mental Health Services https://www.va.gov/health-care/health-needs-conditions/mental-health/

Selections From Staci's "Team Staci F* Cancer Playlist" on Spotify

"Bring on the Rain" by Jo Dee Messina and Tim McGraw
"All She Wants to Do is Dance" by Don Henley
"Angel from Montgomery" by Bonnie Raitt
"Girl on Fire" by Alicia Keys
"Not Ready to Make Nice" by the Chicks
"Roar" by Katy Perry
"Faith" by George Michael
"Walking on Sunshine" by Katrina and the Waves
"Won't Back Down" by Tom Petty
"I'm Still Standing" by Elton John
"Crowded Table" by the Highwomen
"Dreamers" by the Wild Ponies
"Boston Town" by Della Mae
"Unmistakable" by Jo Dee Messina
"Only Girl in the World" by Rihanna
"Follow Your Arrow" by Kacey Musgraves
"Heads Carolina, Tails California" by Jo Dee Messina

ENDNOTES

[1] Joan Didion, *The Year of Magical Thinking* (Alfred A. Knopf, 2005).

[2] Linda Reynolds and Derek Botha, "Anticipatory grief: Its nature, impact, and reasons for contradictory findings," *Counseling, Psychotherapy, and Health* 2, no. 2 (2006): 15–26, https://www.researchgate.net/publication/242079297_Anticipatory_grief_Its_nature_impact_and_reasons_for_contradictory_findings.

[3] Erich Lindemann, "Symptomatology and management of acute grief," *American Journal of Psychiatry* 101, no. 2 (1944): 141–148, doi: 10.1176/ajp.101.2.141.

[4] Elisabeth Kübler-Ross, *On death and dying,* (Macmillan, 1969).

[5] "Kübler-Ross Change Curve," Elisabeth Kübler-Ross Foundation, https://www.ekrfoundation.org/5-stages-of-grief/change-curve/.

[6] Beth Kurland, "For Better Relationships, Get to Know YourNervous System," Psychology Today, March 17, 2022, https://www.psychologytoday.com/us/blog/the-well-being-toolkit/202203/better-relationships-get-know-your-nervous-system.

[7] Tina M. Mason and Allyson R. Duffy, "Complicated Grief and Cortisol Response: An Integrative Review of the Literature," *Journal of the American Psychiatric Nurses Association* 25, no. 3 (2019): 181–188, doi: 10.1177/1078390318807966.

[8] Paul Frysh, "How Grief Can Affect Your Health," WebMD, June 12, 2025, https://www.webmd.com/mental-health/ss/slideshow-grief-health-effects.

[9] Bessel van der Kolk, The Body Keeps the Score: *Brain, Mind, and Body in the Healing of Trauma* (Penguin Books, 2015).

[10] Office of the Surgeon General, "Our Epidemic of Loneliness and Isolation: The U.S. Surgeon General's Advisory on the Healing Effects of Social Connection and Community," *Publication and Reports of the Surgeon General* (2023), https://pubmed.ncbi.nlm.nih.gov/37792968/.

[11] Jared B. Torre and Matthew Lieberman, "Putting Feelings Into Words: Affect Labeling as Implicit Emotion Regulation," *Emotion Review* 10, no. 2 (2018), doi: 10.1177/1754073917742706.

[12] Brianna Abbott, "A New Reality for Terminal Cancer: Longer Lives, With Chronic Uncertainty," *The Wall Street Journal,* August 17, 2025, https://www.wsj.com/health/terminal-cancer-treatments-lifespan-acde24cf?mod=Searchresults&pos=1&page=1.

[13] Marielle Segarra, "Appointment buddy or meal planner? 4 ways to support a friend with cancer," NPR, October 24, 2025, https://www.npr.org/2025/10/24/nx-s1-5464812/not-sure-how-to-support-a-friend-with-cancer-survivors-have-advice.

[14] Marielle Segarra, "Appointment buddy or meal planner? 4 ways to support a friend with cancer," NPR.

[15] Marielle Segarra, "Appointment buddy or meal planner? 4 ways to support a friend with cancer," NPR.

[16] Marielle Segarra, "Appointment buddy or meal planner? 4 ways to support a friend with cancer," NPR.

[17] Marielle Segarra, "Appointment buddy or meal planner? 4 ways to support a friend with cancer," NPR.

[18] Marielle Segarra, "Appointment buddy or meal planner? 4 ways to support a friend with cancer," NPR.

[19] Jim VandeHei, "Axios Finish Line: The power of now," Axios, January 18, 2024, https://www.axios.com/2024/01/19/the-power-of-now.

[20] Jim VandeHei, "Axios Finish Line: The power of now," Axios.

[21] Jim VandeHei, "Axios Finish Line: The power of now," Axios.

[22] "Quick Facts and Statistics About Mental Health," Mental Health America, https://mhanational.org/resources/quick-facts-and-statistics-about-mental-health/.

[23] Mayo Clinic Staff, "Mental health: What's normal, what's not," Mayo Clinic, September 11, 2025, https://www.mayoclinic.org/healthy-lifestyle/adult-health/in-depth/mental-health/art-20044098.

[24] "Sleep and Mood," Division of Sleep Medicine at Harvard Medical School, October 1, 2021, https://sleep.hms.harvard.edu/education-training/public-education/sleep-and-health-education-program/sleep-health-education-87.

[25] Maureen Salamon, "Regular physical activity can boost mood," Harvard Health Publishing, July 1, 2023, https://www.health.harvard.edu/mind-and-mood/regular-physical-activity-can-boost-mood.

[26] "Types of Therapy," Psychology Today, https://www.psychologytoday.com/us/types-of-therapy.

[27] "Yoga for better mental health," Harvard Health Publishing, April 29, 2024, https://www.health.harvard.edu/staying-healthy/yoga-for-better-mental-health.

[28] Tamara Bhandari, "Mind-body connection is built into brain, study suggests," WashU Medicine, https://medicine.washu.edu/news/mind-body-connection-is-built-into-brain-study-suggests/.

[29] Silvia Bellezza, Neeru Paharia, and Anat Keinan, "Research: Why Americans Are So Impressed by Busyness," *Harvard Business Review,* December 15, 2026, https://hbr.org/2016/12/research-why-americans-are-so-impressed-by-busyness.

[30] Adrienne A. Taren et al., "Meditation training alters stress-related amygdala resting state functional connectivity," *Social Cognitive and Affective Neuroscience* 10, no. 12 (2015): 1758–1768, doi: 10.1093/scan/nsv066.

[31] Britta K. Hölzel et al., "Mindfulness practice leads to increases in regional brain gray matter density," *Psychiatry Research: Neuroimaging* 191, no. 1 (2011): 36–43, doi: 10.1016/j.pscychresns.2010.08.006.

[32] Madhav Goyal et al., "Meditation Programs for Psychological Stress and Well-being: A Systematic Review and Meta-analysis," *JAMA Internal Medicine* 174, no. 3 (2014): 357–368, doi: 10.1001/jamainternmed.2013.13018.

[33] Michael I. Norton and Francesca Gino, "Rituals alleviate grieving for loved ones, lovers, and lotteries," *Journal of Experimental Psychology: General* 143, no. 1 (2013): 266–272, doi: 10.1037/a0031772.

[34] Robert A. Neimeyer, "The Language of Loss: Grief Therapy as Meaning Reconstruction," in *Meaning Reconstruction & the Experience of Loss* (American Psychological Association, 2001), 261–292.

[35] Lisa M. Jacola et al., "Longitudinal Assessment of Neurocognitive Outcomes in Survivors of Childhood Acute Lymphoblastic Leukemia Treated on a Contemporary Chemotherapy Protocol," *Journal of Clinical Oncology* 34, no. 11 (2016): 1239–1247, doi: 10.1200/JCO.2015.64.3205.

[36] Michelle C. Janelsins et al., "Longitudinal Changes in Cognitive Function in a Nationwide Cohort Study of Patients With Lymphoma Treated With Chemotherapy," *Journal of the National Cancer Institute* 114, no. 1 (2022): 4759, doi: 10.1093/jnci/djab133.

[37] Erika M. Vitale and Adam S. Smith, "Neurobiology of Loneliness, Isolation, and Loss. Frontiers in Neuroscience," *Frontiers in Behavioral Neuroscience* 16 (2022), doi: 10.3389/fnbeh.2022.846315.

[38] Naomi I. Eisenberger, Matthew D. Lieberman, and Kipling D. Williams, "Does rejection hurt? An FMRI study of social exclusion," *Science* 302, no. 5643 (2003): 290–292, doi: 10.1126/science.1089134.

[39] Naomi I. Eisenberger, "The pain of social disconnection: examining the shared neural underpinnings of physical and

social pain," *Nature Reviews Neuroscience* 13, no. 6 (2012): 421–434, doi: 10.1038/nrn3231.

[40] Caroline Kaercher Kramer and Cristiane Bauermann Leitao, "Laughter as medicine: A systematic review and meta-analysis of interventional studies evaluating the impact of spontaneous laughter on cortisol levels," *PLOS One* 18, no. 5 (2023): e0286260, doi: 10.1371/journal.pone.0286260.

[41] Christopher G. Davis, Susan Nolen-Hoeksema, and Judith Larson, "Making sense of loss and benefiting from the experience: Two construals of meaning," *Journal of Personality and Social Psychology* 75, no. 2 (1998): 561–574, doi: 10.1037/0022-3514.75.2.561.

[42] Robert A. Neimeyer, "Complicated Grief and the Reconstruction of Meaning: Conceptual and Empirical Contributions to a Cognitive-Constructivist Model," *Clinical Psychology: Science and Practice 13*, no. 2 (2006): 141–145, doi: 10.1111/j.1468-2850.2006.00016.x.